Susan Phelan, MHS, MT(ASCP)

Phlebotomy Review Guide

To my husband, Robert (Sonny);
our children, Robert, Meghann, and Christopher;
my parents, Selma and the late William Evers;
and my parents-in-law, Robert (Sonny) and the late Phyllis Phelan

Susan Phelan, MHS, MT(ASCP)

Phlebotomy Review Guide

American Society for
Clinical Pathology
Press

NAACLS does not specifically endorse this or any other phlebotomy curriculum.

American Society for Clinical Pathology Press

Printed in the United States of America

10 09 08 07 10 9 8 7

Contents

Preparing for the Examination

The most time-consuming part of the certification process. The first step in preparing for the examination is to create a study plan. The steps for creating a study plan are as follows:

- Step 1: Establish time in your schedule to study.

  Determine the total number of hours available to you to study for the exam. It is best to budget study time in short sessions, over several weeks. To be most effective, study sessions should not exceed 2 hours in length. To calculate the total number of hours a challenger has to prepare for the exam, the challenger should consult his or her personal calendar and add all of the hours available as study time during the months preceding the exam, to arrive at a total.

- Step 2: Allocate a specific number of hours to each portion of the Content Outline.

  Multiply the total number of hours available for study by the percentages assigned to each topic area listed on the Content Outline. This will segment study time in proportion to the information asked on the exam.

- Step 3: Assign specific areas of study to specific hours on the study schedule.

  Assign the general content areas (Anatomy and Physiology, Specimen Collection, Specimen Processing and Handling, Laboratory Operations) to specific times and days scheduled for study. The total number of hours allocated for each section should equal the number calculated in step 2.

- Step 4: Assign a specific study technique for the study area scheduled.

Assign specific areas (example: venipuncture, skin puncture, etc) to particular dates and times for study. Also, plan a study activity to help you review the material corresponding to that content area. Examples of review activities include: reviewing old notes and quizzes, reviewing chapter objectives and study questions in textbooks, reviewing lab assignments and study questions, and reviewing exam questions in the *Phlebotomy Review Guide*.

Sample Study Plan Worksheet

Step 1: Establish time in your schedule to study.

Most challengers have at least 3 months to prepare for the certification exam of their choice. If there are 4 weeks in a month, and a person studies 12 hours per week, then the total hours allocated to study time would be 144 hours.

Consult your personal calendar and record the total number of hours you can commit to studying for the certification exam in the space provided:

Total number of hours available to study for exam: *___

Step 2: Allocate a specific number of hours to each portion of the Content Outline.

Calculate the number of hours that should be allocated to each portion of the Content Outline.

The Content Outline for the ASCP Exam includes the following percentages:

Anatomy and Physiology	10%
Specimen Collection	50%
Specimen Processing and Handling	20%
Laboratory Operations	20%

Using the 144 hours allocated for the sample study plan, the number of hours that should be assigned to each section is as follows:

Anatomy and Physiology	Specimen Collection	Specimen Processing and Handling	Laboratory Operations
144.0	144.0	144.0	144.0
↔.1	↔.5	↔.2	↔.2
14.4 hours	72.0 hours	28.8 hours	28.8 hours

Therefore, if the challenger allocated 144 total hours to studying for the exam, he or she would spend 14.4 hours on Anatomy and Physiology, 72 hours on Specimen Collection, 28.8 hours on Specimen Processing and Handling, and 28.8 hours on Laboratory Operations.

Calculate the number of hours you can commit to each section, using the operations outlined below. Place the total number of hours you have available to study on the top line of the operations (indicated by an asterisk *). Complete the multiplication. As a result, the number of hours budgeted for each section of the exam will be established, based on the study time you have available.

Anatomy and Physiology	Specimen Collection	Specimen Processing and Handling	Laboratory Operations
*	*	*	*
↔.1 hours	↔.5 hours	↔.2 hours	↔.2 hours

Step 3: Assign specific areas of study to specific hours on the study schedule.

The challenger should outline the study tasks per study day. If the challenger is studying for 2 hour intervals at each study session, his or her plan for the Anatomy and Physiology (A & P) section may look something like this:

Day #1: Structure and Function of the Circulatory System/Heart
Day #2: Structure and Function of the Circulatory System/Arteries, Capillaries, Veins
Day #3: Composition/Types of Blood
Day #4: Composition/Plasma/Serum
Day #5: Composition/Cellular Elements
Day #6: Urine and Other Body Fluids
Day #7: Review all A & P sections

Step 4: Assign a specific study technique for the study area scheduled.

Once again using the A & P section as an example, for each day assigned, a study technique must be specified. For example:

Day #1:
Topic: Structure and Function of the Circulatory System/Heart
Study Technique: Review course objectives, lecture notes, corresponding chapters in course textbooks, and the section related to the structure and function of the heart in *Phlebotomy Review Guide*.

Day #2:
Topic: Structure and Function of the Circulatory System/Arteries, Capillaries, Veins
Study Technique: Review course objectives, lecture notes, corresponding chapters in course textbooks, and the section related to the blood vessels in *Phlebotomy Review Guide*.

Day #3:
Topic: Composition/Types of Blood
Study Technique: Review course objectives, lecture notes, corresponding chapters in course textbooks, and the section related to the types of blood in *Phlebotomy Review Guide*.

Day #4
Topic: Composition/Plasma/Serum
Study Technique: Review course objectives, lecture notes, corresponding chapters in course textbooks, and the section related to the plasma and serum in *Phlebotomy Review Guide*.

Day #5:
Topic: Composition/Cellular Elements
Study Technique: Review course objectives, lecture notes, corresponding chapters in course textbooks, and the section related to the cellular elements of the blood in *Phlebotomy Review Guide*.

Day #6:
Topic: Urine and Other Body Fluids
Study Technique: Review course objectives, lecture notes, corresponding chapters in course textbooks, and the section related to urine and other body fluids in *Phlebotomy Review Guide*.

Day #7:
Topic: Review all A & P sections
Study Technique: Meet with study group. Quiz each other over the A & P section, using *Phlebotomy Review Guide*.

Continue to plan study sessions for the rest of the Content Outline. This is *your study plan*—so individualize it to fit your needs. For example, if you have strong background in the structure and function of the heart, but are weak in the cellular elements of the blood, decrease the time allocated to the study of the heart, and reassign it to studying cellular elements of the blood.

It is important to specify your study techniques as well as content areas. Use the study techniques that have worked best for you in the past. Remember, the sample outlined above is merely an example. Customize the format to fit your needs and study style.

Taking the Exam

Before you take the exam, be sure of the exam site location. Decide on a route and a time line for arriving at the exam site. If necessary, visit the site sometime before you take the test. Determine whether extra money is needed on exam day for tolls, parking, etc. Read the instructions in your test packet, and bring any materials indicated in the packet.

Get a good night's sleep, the night before the exam. Be sure to bring any personal items you may need to the exam site (tissues, watch, throat lozenges). Eat a nutritious meal before the exam. Be sure to speak positively to yourself. Remind yourself that you studied hard during training and clinical, that you were well-organized and diligent in your certification exam study plan, and that you are ready to challenge the exam. It is time to demonstrate what you know!

Before starting the exam, take a few moments to focus your thoughts on the exam. Remove problems, concerns, and negative thoughts from your mind. Take the exam one question at a time. Read the questions and *all of the responses* completely. Select the *best* answer. Keep calm, and methodically proceed through the exam.

Use the checklist below to ensure that you are ready on the day of the exam. Be sure to add anything else you think is important to the list. At the very least, this checklist will help alleviate the “what have I forgotten?” feeling.

__ Reviewed transportation route to examination site

__ Established a time line for arriving at the examination site

__ Money for incidentals (tolls, parking, etc)

__ Additional materials specified in examination packet

__ Personal items (tissues, medications, etc)

__ Nutritious meal

__ Give yourself positive reinforcement (a “pep” talk—from you to you!)

__ Take a few moments to focus your thoughts before starting the exam

Best of luck to you, as you prepare for and challenge your certification examination!

CHAPTER 1

Anatomy and Physiology

1. The body system that functions in calcium storage and hemopoiesis is called the:

   A. digestive system
   B. muscular system
   C. respiratory system
   D. skeletal system

2. The condition where a healthy body through constant changes and functioning remains the same is:

   A. hematoma
   B. hemoconcentration
   C. hemostasis
   D. homeostasis

3. The term for the sum of all chemical reactions necessary to sustain life is:

   A. anabolism
   B. catabolism
   C. embolism
   D. metabolism

4. The process by which complex substances in food are broken down into simple substances while releasing energy is:

   A. anabolism
   B. catabolism
   C. embolism
   D. metabolism

5. The process by which body cells use energy to make complex substances from simpler ones is called:

A. anabolism
B. catabolism
C. embolism
D. metabolism

6. The body plane that runs lengthwise from front to back, dividing the body into right and left halves, is called:

A. frontal plane
B. lateral plane
C. sagittal plane
D. transverse plane

7. The body plane that runs lengthwise from side to side and divides the body into a front and a back half is called:

A. frontal plane
B. proximal plane
C. sagittal plane
D. transverse plane

8. The body plane that runs horizontally, dividing the body into an upper and lower half, is called:

A. frontal plane
B. medial plane
C. sagittal plane
D. transverse plane

9. The directional term that refers to the front of the body is:

A. anterior
B. lateral
C. medial
D. posterior

10. The directional term that refers to the back of the body is:

A. anterior
B. lateral
C. medial
D. posterior

11. The directional term that refers to the front of the body is:

A. dorsal
B. medial
C. posterior
D. ventral

12. The directional term that refers to the back of the body is:

A. dorsal
B. lateral
C. medial
D. ventral

13. The directional term that refers to the midline of the body is:

A. anterior
B. lateral
C. medial
D. posterior

14. The directional term that means toward the side of the body is:

A. anterior
B. lateral
C. medial
D. posterior

15. The directional term that means nearest to the center of the body, point of attachment, or origin is:

A. distal
B. lateral
C. medial
D. proximal

16. The directional term that means farthest from the center of the body, point of attachment, or origin is:

A. distal
B. lateral
C. medial
D. proximal

17. The directional term that means above, higher, or toward the head is:

A. dorsal
B. inferior
C. superior
D. ventral

18. The directional term that means lower, beneath, or away from the head is:

A. dorsal
B. inferior
C. superior
D. ventral

19. The directional term that means higher or toward the head is:

A. caudal
B. cranial
C. lateral
D. medial

20. The directional term that means lower or away from the head is:

A. caudal
B. cranial
C. dorsal
D. ventral

21. If a person is lying on the back, that person is said to be in which of the following positions?

A. anatomic
B. distal
C. proximal
D. supine

22. If a person is standing erect, with palms facing forward, he or she is in what position?

A. anatomic
B. distal
C. proximal
D. supine

23. Which of the following body cavities is located in the back of the body?

A. abdominal
B. cranial
C. pelvic
D. thoracic

24. Which of the following body cavities are located in the front of the body?

A. abdominal
B. cranial
C. dorsal
D. spinal

25. The body cavity that houses the brain is the:

A. abdominal cavity
B. cranial cavity
C. pelvic cavity
D. thoracic cavity

26. The body cavity that houses the heart and the lungs is the:

A. abdominal cavity
B. cranial cavity
C. spinal cavity
D. thoracic cavity

27. The body cavity that houses the stomach, liver, pancreas, gallbladder, and spleen is the:

A. abdominal cavity
B. pelvic cavity
C. spinal cavity
D. thoracic cavity

28. The body cavity that houses the urinary bladder and the reproductive organs is the:

A. abdominal cavity
B. cranial cavity
C. pelvic cavity
D. thoracic cavity

29. Which of the following blood vessels has the thickest vessel wall?

A. arteries
B. arterioles
C. capillaries
D. veins

30. Which of the following structures is located on the sagittal plane?

A. intestines
B. left kidney
C. right lung
D. sternum

31. Which of the following structures is located on the posterior side of the frontal plane?

A. bladder
B. diaphragm
C. epididymis
D. spinal cord

32. Which of the following structures is located inferior to the transverse plane?

A. brain
B. heart
C. lungs
D. uterus

33. The cellular elements of the blood responsible for the transport of oxygen to the tissues are called:

A. erythrocytes
B. leukocytes
C. megakaryocytes
D. thrombocytes

34. The cellular elements of the blood that function in coagulation are called:

A. erythrocyte
B. leukocyte
C. macrophage
D. thrombocyte

35. The cellular elements of the blood that function in fighting infection are called:

A. erythrocytes
B. leukocytes
C. megakaryocytes
D. thrombocytes

36. Granulocytes that function in fighting bacterial infection are called:

A. eosinophilic segmented cells
B. neutrophilic segmented cells
C. lymphocytes
D. monocytes

37. Agranulocytes that function in antibody production are called:

A. eosinophilic segmented cells
B. neutrophilic segmented cells
C. lymphocytes
D. monocytes

38. What is the fluid portion of a blood specimen called after the specimen has been collected into an anticoagulant?

A. fibrin
B. fibrinogen
C. plasma
D. serum

39. Which of the following is found in plasma, but not in serum?

A. fibrinogen
B. prothrombin
C. thrombin
D. tissue thromboplastin

40. The process by which the body stops the leakage of blood from the vascular system is called:

A. hematoma
B. hemoconcentration
C. hemostasis
D. homeostasis

41. What are the three components of coagulation?

A. blood vessels, coagulation factors, platelets
B. blood vessels, platelets, fibrin
C. platelets, fibrin, serum
D. fibrinogen, prothrombin, antihemophilic factor

42. Which of the following pathways is initiated through the activation of factor XII?

A. extrinsic pathway
B. intrinsic pathway
C. common pathway
D. fibrinolytic pathway

43. Which of the following pathways is initiated by the release of tissue thromboplastin?

A. extrinsic pathway
B. intrinsic pathway
C. common pathway
D. fibrinolytic pathway

44. The pathway that is initiated by the intrinsic and extrinsic pathways is the:

A. common pathway
B. complement cascade
C. fibrinolytic pathway
D. hemostatic plug

45. Fibrin degradation products are the end result of the:

A. intrinsic pathway
B. extrinsic pathway
C. common pathway
D. fibrinolytic pathway

46. The body system that provides communication in the body by means of electrical impulses and chemical substances is the:

A. digestive system
B. muscular system
C. nervous system
D. respiratory system

47. The body system that functions to maintain posture and produce heat is the:

A. digestive system
B. muscular system
C. respiratory system
D. skeletal system

48. The body system that mechanically and chemically breaks down food into nutrients that can be absorbed and used by the body's cells is the:

A. digestive system
B. endocrine system
C. muscular system
D. skeletal system

49. The body system that functions in ovulation, labor, and pregnancy is the:

A. endocrine system
B. female reproductive system
C. male reproductive system
D. urinary system

50. The body system responsible for eliminating metabolic waste products from the body is the:

A. endocrine system
B. female reproductive system
C. male reproductive system
D. urinary system

51. The body system responsible for delivering air to the capillary beds surrounding the alveoli is the:

A. endocrine system
B. integumentary system
C. respiratory system
D. urinary system

52. The glandular system that secretes hormones directly into the bloodstream is the:

A. endocrine system
B. exocrine system
C. integumentary system
D. respiratory system

53. The blood vessel whose wall is one cell layer thick is the:

A. arteriole
B. artery
C. capillary
D. vein

54. The blood vessels that have valves are the:

A. arterioles
B. arteries
C. capillaries
D. veins

55. The blood vessels with the largest tunica media are the:

A. arterioles
B. arteries
C. capillaries
D. veins

56. The blood vessels that carry blood away from the heart are the:

A. arteries
B. capillaries
C. vena cava
D. veins

57. The four-chambered, muscular organ that pumps blood through the circulatory system is the:

A. brain
B. heart
C. pancreas
D. stomach

58. Oxygenated blood is found in which of the following blood vessels?

A. arteries
B. pulmonary arteries
C. veins
D. venules

59. Deoxygenated blood is found in which of the following blood vessels?

A. arteries
B. arterioles
C. pulmonary veins
D. veins

60. After performing a routine venipuncture, the phlebotomist noticed that the blood in the evacuated tube was bright cherry red. What vessel did the phlebotomist puncture?

A. artery
B. pulmonary artery
C. capillary
D. vein

61. The body fluid that may be extracted from a joint cavity is called:

A. cerebrospinal fluid
B. pleural fluid
C. peritoneal fluid
D. synovial fluid

62. The body fluid that may be removed from between the parietal and visceral membranes of the lungs is called:

A. cerebrospinal fluid
B. pleural fluid
C. peritoneal fluid
D. synovial fluid

63. The clear, colorless fluid that functions in protecting and nourishing the brain and spinal cord is called:

A. ascitic fluid
B. CSF
C. pericardial fluid
D. synovial fluid

64. The abnormal accumulation of serous fluid is called:

A. effusion
B. exudate
C. transudate
D. paracentesis

65. Blood exits the heart from the right atrium through which of the following valves?

A. aortic valve
B. mitral valve
C. pulmonic valve
D. tricuspid valve

66. Blood exits the heart from the left ventricle through which of the following valves?

A. aortic
B. mitral
C. pulmonic
D. tricuspid

67. Blood enters the right side of the heart from which of the following blood vessels?

A. aorta
B. pulmonary artery
C. pulmonary vein
D. superior vena cava

68. Blood enters the left side of the heart through which of the following blood vessels?

A. aorta
B. pulmonary artery
C. pulmonary vein
D. superior vena cava

69. Which of the following structures contains deoxygenated blood?

A. aorta
B. left atrium
C. left ventricle
D. right atrium

70. Which of the following structures contains oxygenated blood?

A. aorta
B. right atrium
C. right ventricle
D. superior vena cava

71. Which of the following structures is included in the pulmonary circuit?

A. aorta
B. coronary artery
C. pulmonary artery
D. right atrium

72. Which of the following structures is a part of the systemic circuit?

A. aorta
B. pulmonary artery
C. right atrium
D. right ventricle

CHAPTER 2

Specimen Collection

73. A term that means "syringe" is:

A. evacuated blood collection system
B. nonevacuated blood collection system
C. Microtainer™
D. Unopette™

74. Specimens for which of the following tests must be collected by syringe?

A. ABG
B. BUN
C. CBC
D. ESR

75. On which of the following patients would a phlebotomist most likely choose a syringe to perform a venipuncture?

A. a 14-year-old high school freshman
B. a 46-year-old high school teacher
C. a 53-year-old construction worker
D. an 85-year-old grandmother

76. On which of the following patients would a phlebotomist most likely use a syringe to collect a blood specimen?

A. a woman who had a mastectomy
B. a man with a heparin lock
C. a woman who just suffered a miscarriage
D. a man who just underwent angioplasty surgery

77. The closed system that is composed of a needle, a holder, and a tube containing a premeasured amount of vacuum is the:

A. evacuated blood collection system
B. nonevacuated blood collection system
C. Microtainer™ system
D. Unopette™ system

78. Which of the following needle lengths is most commonly used for adult venipuncture?

A. 1/2 and 1 inch needles
B. 1 and 1-1/2 inch needles
C. 1-1/2 and 2 inch needles
D. 2 and 2-1/2 inch needles

79. What criterion does a phlebotomist use when selecting needle gauge prior to a venipuncture procedure?

A. if the specimen is arterial or venous
B. direction of the patient's vein
C. the lumen size of the patient's vein
D. the physician's order

80. Evacuated tubes are manufactured in a range of sizes. Which of the range of volumes listed below most accurately reflects available sizes of evacuated tubes?

A. 1 to 15 mL
B. 1 to 25 mL
C. 2 to 20 mL
D. 2 to 30 mL

81. An evacuated tube contains clot activator and serum separator gel. What color is the Hemogard™ closure?

A. gold
B. green
C. light green
D. royal blue

82. An evacuated tube contains thrombin. What color is the Hemogard™ closure?

A. gold
B. green
C. orange
D. royal blue

83. If an evacuated tube contains heparin and plasma separator gel, what color is the Hemogard™ closure?

A. gold
B. light green
C. orange
D. royal blue

84. Which of the following blood collection devices is manufactured with a rubber sheath?

A. single sample needle
B. multisample needle
C. evacuated tube
D. nonevacuated tube

85. Which of the following additives is found in a red stoppered evacuated tube?

A. EDTA
B. SPS
C. none
D. sodium heparin

86. Which of the following additives is found in an evacuated tube with a green conventional stopper?

A. EDTA
B. SPS
C. none
D. sodium heparin

87. Which of the following additives is found in an evacuated tube with a gray conventional stopper?

A. EDTA
B. SPS
C. sodium citrate
D. sodium fluoride

88. Which of the following additives is found in an evacuated tube with a yellow conventional stopper?

A. EDTA
B. SPS
C. sodium citrate
D. sodium fluoride

89. Which of the following additives in evacuated tubes binds calcium?

A. sodium heparin
B. potassium oxalate
C. sodium citrate
D. thrombin

90. Which of the following additives in evacuated tubes neutralizes thrombin?

A. ACD
B. EDTA
C. sodium heparin
D. sodium citrate

91. Which of the following evacuated tube stoppers is manufactured with the lowest verified levels of trace elements available?

A. lavender
B. light blue
C. royal blue
D. yellow

92. Which of the following evacuated tube stoppers is manufactured with very low levels of lead?

A. tan
B. lavender
C. red
D. red SST

93. Which of the following additives is found in lavender stoppered evacuated tubes?

A. ACD
B. CPDA
C. EDTA
D. SPS

94. Which of the following additives is found in an evacuated tube with a yellow conventional stopper?

A. ACD
B. EDTA
C. lithium heparin
D. sodium citrate

95. Which of the following additives is found in an evacuated tube with a light blue conventional stopper?

A. ACD
B. EDTA
C. lithium heparin
D. sodium citrate

96. Which of the following additives in evacuated tubes binds calcium?

A. EDTA
B. potassium oxalate
C. sodium heparin
D. thrombin

97. Which of the following additives in evacuated tubes promotes clotting?

A. ACD
B. EDTA
C. heparin
D. thrombin

98. The standard for measuring the diameter of the lumen of a needle is the needle:

A. bore
B. brand
C. gauge
D. length

99. The internal space of a needle is the needle's:

A. bevel
B. brand
C. gauge
D. lumen

100. Which of the following needles has the largest interior diameter?

A. 18
B. 19
C. 20
D. 21

101. Which of the following needles has the smallest interior diameter?

A. 20
B. 21
C. 22
D. 23

102. Listed below are conventional stopper colors of evacuated tubes. Which stopper color should be used when collecting specimens for analyses that require *both* a patient's cells and serum?

A. green
B. green PST
C. red
D. red SST

103. Listed below are conventional stopper colors of evacuated tubes. Which stopper color indicates the tube contains silica particles to facilitate blood clotting?

A. red
B. red SST
C. green
D. green PST

104. Which of the following needle gauges is used most often to perform routine venipuncture?

A. 20 and 21
B. 21 and 22
C. 22 and 23
D. 23 and 24

105. Which of the following additives in evacuated tubes acts as a glycolytic inhibitor?

A. lithium heparin
B. potassium oxalate
C. sodium citrate
D. sodium fluoride

106. Which of the following additives in evacuated tubes prevents platelets from clumping?

A. EDTA
B. SPS
C. potassium oxalate
D. sodium citrate

107. Which of the following additives in evacuated tubes preserves labile coagulation factors?

A. EDTA
B. SPS
C. sodium citrate
D. sodium heparin

108. Which of the following additives in evacuated tubes produces artifact residue on blood smears stained with Wright's stain?

A. EDTA
B. fibrin
C. sodium heparin
D. thrombin

109. A phlebotomist transfixes a vein during venipuncture. Which of the following specimen characteristics may result?

A. clotting in plasma tubes
B. hemolyzed specimen
C. hemoconcentration of specimen
D. short draw

110. A phlebotomist obtains a specimen from a patient, following a traumatized venipuncture. Which of the following specimen characteristics may result?

A. hemoconcentration
B. hemolysis
C. glycolysis
D. lipemia

111. A lavender stoppered evacuated tube must be redrawn because of clots in the tube. What collection error causes this?

A. traumatized specimen
B. transfixed vein
C. improper patient preparation
D. insufficient mixing of additive with specimen

112. Which of the following equipment would a phlebotomist carry on his or her tray for a skin puncture procedure?

A. holder, needle, evacuated tube
B. syringe, heparin, ice
C. Simplate™ , filter paper, stopwatch
D. lancet, Microtainer™ , gauze

113. A potential complication of accidentally puncturing the calcaneus bone during skin puncture, characterized by inflammation of the bone and bone marrow, is called:

A. osteocarcinoma
B. osteochondritis
C. osteomyelitis
D. osteoporosis

114. A potential complication of accidentally puncturing the calcaneus bone during skin puncture, characterized by inflammation of the bone and cartilage, is called:

A. osteocarcinoma
B. osteochondritis
C. osteomyelitis
D. osteoporosis

115. A potential complication of accidentally puncturing the calcaneus bone during skin puncture, characterized by the presence of pathogenic microorganisms or their toxins in the blood or other tissues, is called:

A. osteochondritis
B. osteomyelitis
C. sepsis
D. stasis

116. An inherited condition that is caused by the body's inability to metabolize phenylalanine is called:

A. PCV
B. PID
C. PKU
D. PPLO

117. Which of the following values are higher in newborns than in adults?

A. electrolyte levels
B. red cell counts
C. heterophile titer levels
D. varicella zoster virus

118. Which of the following blood constituents will increase as the oxygen content of the air decreases?

A. red blood cell counts
B. white blood cell counts
C. CK levels
D. LDH levels

119. Which of the following values are higher in the morning?

A. cortisol levels
B. eosinophil counts
C. iron levels
D. WBC counts

120. Eating which of the following foods can cause lipemic serum in a patient's blood specimen?

A. apple
B. butter
C. carrot
D. hard candy

121. Which of the following can affect cortisol levels?

A. caffeine
B. glucose
C. lipids
D. saccharin

122. Which of the following levels will remain elevated for at least 24 hours following exercise?

A. ABG
B. BUN
C. CBC
D. CK

123. A patient is being treated with a thiazide diuretic. Which health care professional is responsible for recognizing potential drug interferences with test results?

A. medical technologist
B. nurse
C. phlebotomist
D. physician

124. Changing a patient's position from supine to standing will cause which physiologic change?

A. no change will occur
B. plasma glucose will increase
C. water will filter from the plasma to the tissues
D. water will filter from the tissues to the plasma

125. During pregnancy, the increase of body fluids may cause a patient's RBC count to:

A. decrease
B. increase
C. remain unchanged
D. show no difference due to gender

126. Which of the following patient conditions may cause a transient elevation in WBC count results?

A. altitude change
B. gender
C. pregnancy
D. stress

127. A new field of medicine that deals with the study of interaction between the brain, endocrine system, and the immune system is called:

A. psychiatry
B. psychoneuroimmunology
C. psychoanaleptic
D. psychodometry

128. What method of blood collection is preferred for infants?

A. accessing indwelling lines
B. arterial puncture
C. skin puncture
D. venipuncture

129. Specimens for home glucose monitoring are routinely collected by:

A. accessing indwelling lines
B. arterial puncture
C. skin puncture
D. venipuncture

130. Specimens for which of the following patients should be drawn by skin puncture?

A. a new admit, for a chemistry profile
B. a 6-month-old baby for a blood culture
C. a 25-year-old woman for type and crossmatch
D. an oncology patient, for a WBC count and platelet count

131. Why is skin puncture preferred over venipuncture for infants for the collection of blood specimens?

A. continuous quality indicator
B. increased accuracy of test results
C. prevent anemia
D. prevent infection

132. Which of the following tests is most commonly performed on skin puncture samples?

A. PCV
B. pH
C. PKU
D. PTT

133. Which of the following collection procedures will yield a specimen composed of arterial, venous, and capillary blood?

A. arterial puncture
B. drawing from an indwelling line
C. skin puncture
D. venipuncture

134. If a skin puncture site is warmed prior to blood collection, the specimen is said to be:

A. arterialized
B. concentrated
C. hemolyzed
D. ischemic

135. Which of the following test procedures *cannot* be performed on specimens collected by skin puncture?

A. bilirubin
B. blood cultures
C. calcium
D. T3, T4

136. Which of the following test procedures *cannot* be performed on specimens collected by skin puncture?

A. bilirubin
B. calcium
C. ESR
D. T3, T4

137. Which of the following test procedures *cannot* be performed on specimens collected by skin puncture?

A. APTT
B. bilirubin
C. calcium
D. T3, T4

138. Which of the following information should *not* be provided to the patient by the phlebotomist?

A. if the phlebotomist is a student
B. the department the phlebotomist works in
C. the phlebotomist's name
D. what the test is for

139. Which of the following laboratory professionals has the greatest public relations responsibility for the laboratory?

A. pathologist
B. phlebotomist
C. medical laboratory technician
D. medical technologist

140. A phlebotomist enters a patient's room at 5:30 AM, but the patient is asleep. The phlebotomist should:

A. ask the nurse to wake the patient
B. gently wake the patient and proceed
C. mark the slip "Can't get," and return to the lab
D. return to the patient's room later

141. A phlebotomist is about to collect a blood specimen from a patient in ICU, but the patient is unconscious. The phlebotomist should:

A. call a code
B. call a nurse
C. proceed as though the patient were conscious
D. return when the patient awakens

142. Which of the following personnel has priority with the patient?

A. phlebotomist with a stat request
B. physician talking to a patient
C. nurse giving the patient a bed bath
D. respiratory therapist

143. Which of the following personnel has priority with the patient?

A. clergyman administering Communion
B. nurse giving a bed bath
C. phlebotomist to collect a CBC
D. respiratory therapist

144. If a patient is not in his or her room, how should the phlebotomist locate the patient?

A. ask at the nurse's station
B. page the patient
C. refer to the patient's chart
D. search the laboratory's computer

145. If a patient's family is in the patient's room when the phlebotomist enters, the phlebotomist should:

A. ask the family to restrain the patient
B. ask the family to step outside the room
C. explain the test's clinical significance
D. ignore the family

146. How many steps are involved in proper patient identification?

A. 1
B. 2
C. 3
D. 4

147. What is the first step in proper patient identification?

A. the phlebotomist asks, "Are you Mrs. Smith?"
B. the nurse identifies the patient by room number
C. the patient is asked to state his or her name
D. the phlebotomist reads the card above the bed

148. What is the most important step in patient identification?

A. asking "Are you Mrs. Smith?"
B. verifying identification with the nurse
C. verifying identification with a visitor
D. comparing the medical record number on the requisition with the patient's wristband

149. Which of the following information should NEVER be the same on any two patients?

A. date of birth
B. first names
C. last names
D. medical record number

150. If a patient's wristband matches the requisition entirely except for the medical record number, the phlebotomist should:

A. change the number on the requisition
B. change the number on the wristband
C. contact the nurse's station
D. draw the patient

151. If a patient's identification bracelet is on his or her nightstand and it matches the requisition exactly, the phlebotomist should:

A. ask a nurse to affix the wristband on the patient
B. discard the requisition
C. discard the wristband
D. draw the patient

152. What infection control equipment should the phlebotomist use when performing a skin puncture procedure?

A. alcohol, sterile gauze
B. heel warmer, Unopette™ , Simplate™
C. lancet, capillary tubes, heel warmer, alcohol pad
D. sharps, biohazard bag, gown, gloves

153. What equipment does the phlebotomist need for site preparation prior to skin puncture?

A. heel warmer, alcohol, sterile gauze
B. heel warmer, povidone iodine, sterile gauze
C. lancet, Unopette™ , sharps, gloves
D. gown, gloves, sharps, biohazard bag

154. Heel warmers should heat within which of the following temperature ranges?

A. 35° to 39°C
B. 36° to 40°C
C. 37° to 41°C
D. 39° to 42°C

155. What is the maximum length lancet that may be safely used for skin puncture on an infant's foot?

A. 2.4 mm
B. 3.0 mm
C. 2.4 cm
D. 3.0 cm

156. Which of the following describes the best site to select for skin puncture on an infant's foot?

A. arch area of the foot
B. lateral portion of the palmar surface of the heel
C. lateral portion of the plantar surface of the heel
D. posterior curvature of the heel

157. Which of the following sites is acceptable to use for skin puncture on an infant's foot?

A. arch of the foot
B. lateral portion of the palmar surface of the heel
C. posterior curvature of the heel
D. the great toe

158. Which of the following describes the best site to select for skin puncture, using a patient's finger?

A. distal phalanx of the index finger
B. distal phalanx of the little finger
C. distal phalanx of the middle finger
D. distal phalanx of the thumb

159. Which of the following sites is the best site to select for skin puncture, using a patient's finger?

A. distal phalanx of the index finger
B. distal phalanx of the little finger
C. distal phalanx of the ring finger
D. distal phalanx of the thumb

160. Which of the following sites is the best site to select for skin puncture, using a patient's finger?

A. distal phalanx of the thumb, palmar surface
B. index finger, palmar surface
C. little finger, palmar surface
D. middle finger, palmar surface

161. Skin punctures performed on patients' fingers should be made:

A. at the crease between the first and second phalanx
B. on the very tip of the finger
C. parallel to the fingerprints
D. perpendicular to the fingerprints

162. If a heel warmer is applied to a skin puncture site, this will:

A. decrease blood flow to the site
B. increase blood flow to the site
C. prevent hemoconcentration of the specimen
D. prevent hemolysis of the specimen

163. By how much can blood flow to a skin puncture site be increased if a warmer is applied prior to skin puncture?

A. 4 times
B. 5 times
C. 6 times
D. 7 times

164. What portion of the capillary circulation is increased when a warmer is applied to a skin puncture site?

A. arterial
B. capillary
C. interstitial fluid
D. venous

165. At least how long should a warmer be applied to a skin puncture site prior to making a skin puncture?

A. 3 minutes
B. 4 minutes
C. 5 minutes
D. 6 minutes

166. Which of the following tests *requires* that the site be warmed prior to skin puncture?

A. bilirubin
B. calcium
C. capillary blood gases
D. reticulocyte count

167. Which of the following actions may result in a QNS skin puncture specimen?

A. alcohol contamination
B. anemic condition of the patient
C. failure to wipe away the first drop of blood
D. insufficient puncture

168. What is the rationale for the order of draw for the collection of multiple specimens following skin puncture?

A. minimize contamination
B. minimize hemoconcentration
C. minimize hemolysis
D. minimize platelet clumping

169. The following tests were to be collected from a patient following skin puncture: platelet count, bilirubin, T3. In what order should these tests be collected?

A. bilirubin, platelet count, T3
B. bilirubin, T3, platelet count
C. platelet count, bilirubin, T3
D. T3, bilirubin, platelet count

170. The following Microtainers™ were to be collected following skin puncture: lavender, pink, red SST. In what order should the microtainers be collected?

A. lavender, pink, red SST
B. pink, red SST, lavender
C. pink, lavender, red SST
D. red SST, lavender, pink

171. What is the maximum number of times an infant's heel may be punctured to collect a blood specimen?

A. 1
B. 2
C. 3
D. 4

172. Which of the following could cause hemolysis of a specimen obtained by skin puncture?

A. collecting specimens in an incorrect order
B. residual alcohol left on the site
C. using povidone iodine to clean the site
D. warming the site

173. Which of the following could cause hemolysis of a specimen collected by skin puncture?

A. excessive squeezing of the puncture site to secure the specimen
B. incorrect order of draw
C. using povidone iodine to prepare the site
D. warming the site

174. Bleeding time procedures are usually ordered:

A. as timed tests
B. in a series
C. presurgically
D. stat

175. Bleeding times are used to assess which of the following?

A. coumarin dosage
B. fibrinogen levels
C. heparin dosage
D. platelet function

176. Bleeding times are used to assess which of the following?

A. blood vessel integrity
B. pancreatic function
C. risk of diabetes
D. risk of heart disease

177. Which of the following can influence the results of a bleeding time test?

A. cholesterol level
B. circulating von Willebrand's factor
C. glucose level
D. potassium level

178. Which of the following medications will interfere with the bleeding time test result?

A. acetaminophen
B. aspirin
C. insulin
D. furosemide

179. Which of the following medications will interfere with the results of the bleeding time test?

A. acetaminophen
B. insulin
C. furosemide
D. salicylic acid

180. Before starting a bleeding time test, the phlebotomist should:

A. ask the patient to sign a consent form
B. ask the patient if he or she has eaten
C. ask the patient if he or she has taken any medications
D. take the patient's blood pressure

181. Which of the following procedures is routinely performed on a patient's earlobe?

A. Duke bleeding time
B. glucose tolerance test
C. lactose tolerance test
D. modified Ivy bleeding time

182. Which of the following is used to collect blood following the puncture in a Duke bleeding time procedure?

A. filter paper
B. microhematocrit tube
C. Microtainer™ tube
D. Unopette™

183. Which of the following compounds is used to prepare the site prior to the puncture in a Duke bleeding time procedure?

A. alcohol
B. heel warmer
C. ice
D. iodine

184. During a Duke bleeding time procedure, a phlebotomist touches the wound with the collection device. The bleeding time results will be:

A. falsely decreased
B. falsely prolonged
C. impossible to interpret
D. unchanged

185. If a patient has taken aspirin, how long will it affect the patient's platelet function?

A. 1 to 2 hours
B. 7 to 10 minutes
C. 1 to 2 days
D. 7 to 10 days

186. If a test procedure can be performed the same way, on the same patient, and generate almost identical results, the test is said to be:

A. reliable
B. reproducible
C. sensitive
D. specific

187. A test that will detect borderline abnormalities in a patient is said to be:

A. reproducible
B. reliable
C. sensitive
D. specific

188. If a physician wishes to assess a patient's platelet function, which of the following tests will provide the physician with the most reliable results?

A. capillary bleeding time
B. Duke bleeding time
C. modified Ivy bleeding time
D. tourniquet test

189. If a physician would like to screen platelet function in a patient, which of the following tests will provide the physician with the most sensitive results?

A. capillary bleeding time
B. Duke bleeding time
C. modified Ivy bleeding time
D. tourniquet test

190. Why is the Duke bleeding time procedure not routinely performed in modern medical practice?

A. dangerous collection container
B. lack of standardized puncture
C. too many patient complaints
D. too messy

191. The use of a template and surgical incision as part of a bleeding time procedure was first introduced by:

A. Duke
B. Ivy
C. Landsteiner
D. Mielke

192. What equipment should a phlebotomist carry on his or her tray for the Ivy bleeding time procedure?

A. bleeding time device, alcohol
B. bleeding time device, iodine
C. steel blade lancet, alcohol
D. steel blade lancet, iodine

193. What equipment should a phlebotomist carry on his or her tray for an Ivy bleeding time procedure?

A. bleeding time device, blood pressure cuff
B. blood pressure cuff, iodine
C. filter paper, steel blade lancet
D. iodine, filter paper

194. What equipment should a phlebotomist carry on his or her tray for an Ivy bleeding time procedure?

A. bleeding time device, iodine
B. filter paper, steel blade lancet
C. butterfly bandage, blood pressure cuff
D. butterfly bandage, iodine

195. The Ivy bleeding time procedure is routinely performed on the patient's:

A. earlobe
B. foot
C. forearm
D. wrist

196. The Ivy bleeding time procedure is routinely performed on the patient's:

A. distal phalanx of the ring finger, palmar surface
B. lateral area of the plantar surface of the foot
C. lateral aspect, volar surface of the forearm
D. medial area of the plantar surface of the foot

197. During an Ivy bleeding time procedure, the blood pressure cuff should be positioned:

A. above the antecubital crease
B. below the antecubital crease
C. around the patient's calf
D. around the patient's wrist

198. During an Ivy bleeding time procedure, the blood pressure cuff should be inflated to:

A. 35 mm Hg
B. 40 mm Hg
C. 45 mm Hg
D. 50 mm Hg

199. During an Ivy bleeding time procedure, the maximum length of time that may elapse between inflation of the blood pressure cuff and making the incision is:

A. 10 seconds
B. 60 seconds
C. 90 seconds
D. 120 seconds

200. The dimensions of the most commonly used bleeding time devices are:

A. 1 mm deep × 3 mm wide
B. 1 mm deep × 5 mm wide
C. 3 mm deep × 5 mm wide
D. 5 mm deep × 1 mm wide

201. During an Ivy bleeding time procedure, the phlebotomist should start the stopwatch:

A. after applying the tourniquet
B. after blotting the first drop of blood
C. simultaneously with the incision
D. when the blood pressure cuff is applied

202. A potential patient complication of the Ivy bleeding time test is:

A. hematoma
B. scarring
C. poor reproducibility
D. poor sensitivity

203. Two examples of bleeding time devices are:

A. Safety flow lancet™ , steel blade lancet
B. Simplate™ , Surgicutt™
C. Microtainer™ and Unopette™
D. Unopette™ and Tenderfoot™

204. Cleaning the bleeding time puncture site too vigorously may cause:

A. hemoconcentration
B. hemolysis
C. hyperemia
D. hyperchromia

205. What effect will increasing blood flow to the bleeding time site have on the results of the procedure?

A. falsely decreased
B. falsely elevated
C. impossible to predict
D. no effect

206. What effect will dislodging the platelet plug have on bleeding time results?

A. falsely decreased
B. falsely elevated
C. impossible to predict
D. no effect

207. During an Ivy bleeding time procedure, which position of the bleeding time device offers a cosmetic advantage to the patient?

A. parallel to the antecubital crease
B. perpendicular to the antecubital crease
C. tilted to the left of the phlebotomist
D. tilted to the right of the phlebotomist

208. During an Ivy bleeding time procedure, which position of the bleeding time device is more sensitive to borderline abnormalities?

A. parallel to the antecubital crease
B. perpendicular to the antecubital crease
C. tilted to the left of the phlebotomist
D. tilted to the right of the phlebotomist

209. Prior to making a puncture during a blood collection procedure, antiseptic solution should be applied to the site selected:

A. in concentric circles, beginning at the puncture site
B. in concentric circles, beginning away from the puncture site
C. parallel to the antecubital crease
D. perpendicular to the antecubital crease

210. To examine by touch or feel is to:

A. palate
B. palpitate
C. palpate
D. patency

211. A return flow of blood from an evacuated tube into a patient's arm during a venipuncture procedure is called:

A. reflex
B. reflux
C. reagent
D. refractile

212. Small, nonraised bruises the size of a pinpoint are called:

A. patella
B. pedicel
C. petechiae
D. pellicle

213. The condition in which the fluid portion of the blood filters into the tissues, decreasing the fluid portion of the blood in the blood vessels, is called:

A. hemochromoprotein
B. hemoclastic
C. hemoconcentration
D. hemocuprein

214. The liberation of hemoglobin into the plasma following destruction of red blood cells is called:

A. hemagglutination
B. hemoconcentration
C. hemolysis
D. hemostasis

215. What is the medical term for the following symptoms: dizziness, pallor, sweating, clammy skin, unconsciousness?

A. emesis
B. hematoma
C. syncope
D. tetany

216. The accumulation of fluid in the tissues is called:

A. edema
B. emesis
C. syncope
D. tetany

217. Under universal precautions, what PPE must the phlebotomist use for every blood collection procedure?

A. gloves
B. gown
C. gown, gloves, sharps, and biohazard bag
D. sharps and biohazard bag

218. To prepare a puncture site prior to routine venipuncture, the phlebotomist would use:

A. 50% isopropyl alcohol
B. 70% isopropyl alcohol
C. betadine
D. povidone iodine

219. Which of the following equipment is used for a routine venipuncture?

A. heel warmer, lancet, Microtainer™
B. heel warmer, needle, Microtainer™
C. needle, evacuated tube, holder
D. syringe, evacuated tube

220. Which of the following equipment is used for site selection and preparation during routine skin puncture?

A. betadine
B. povidone iodine
C. heel warmer
D. tourniquet

221. What is the correct sequence of the following steps in a routine venipuncture procedure?

A. apply alcohol, palpate site, apply tourniquet
B. apply tourniquet, palpate site, release tourniquet
C. palpate site, apply alcohol, apply tourniquet
D. palpate site, apply tourniquet, apply alcohol

222. What is the correct sequence of the following steps in a routine venipuncture procedure?

A. anchor the vein, insert the needle, uncap the needle
B. anchor the vein, uncap the needle, insert the needle
C. uncap the needle, anchor the vein, insert the needle
D. uncap the needle, insert the needle, anchor the vein

223. During routine venipuncture, the needle should be inserted:

A. bevel down
B. bevel up
C. bevel turned toward the left
D. bevel turned toward the right

224. During routine venipuncture, needles should be inserted at which of the following angles, relative to the patient's arm?

A. 0 to 10 degrees
B. 5 to 10 degrees
C. 15 to 30 degrees
D. 30 to 45 degrees

225. During routine venipuncture, how should the needle be positioned, relative to the vein selected?

A. perpendicular
B. parallel, 1 inch below
C. parallel, 1 inch above
D. same direction

226. During routine venipuncture, how deep should the needle be inserted?

A. 1 inch
B. 1-1/2 inch
C. until the phlebotomist feels a slight decrease in resistance
D. until the phlebotomist feels a slight increase in resistance

227. What is the correct sequence of the following steps in a routine venipuncture procedure?

A. release tourniquet, engage tube, release vein
B. release tourniquet, release the vein, engage the tube
C. release vein, engage tube, release tourniquet
D. release vein, release tourniquet, engage tube

228. During venipuncture, the tourniquet should be left on a patient's arm no longer than:

A. 1 to 2 minutes
B. 2 to 3 minutes
C. 3 to 4 minutes
D. 4 to 5 minutes

229. A patient has undergone a left radical mastectomy. Which site *cannot* be used for venipuncture until the patient's physician is consulted?

A. cephalic hand vein
B. dorsal hand vein
C. left arm
D. right arm

230. What condition sometimes occurs following mastectomy that becomes a factor in venipuncture site selection?

A. hemostasis
B. homeostasis
C. lymphostasis
D. venous stasis

231. The phlebotomist inspects the antecubital fossa of a patient and notes that the area surrounding the puncture site is purple, accompanied by swelling of the puncture site. What is the name of this condition?

A. hematoma
B. hemangioma
C. lipoma
D. lymphoma

232. If a phlebotomist notes a purple swelling around the site selected for venipuncture, he or she should:

A. notify the nurse
B. proceed, using the site selected
C. select another site
D. write "Can't get" on the requisition

233. What condition, caused by a hematoma surrounding a venipuncture site, may lead to erroneous results?

A. hemostasis
B. homeostasis
C. lymphostasis
D. venous stasis

234. Swelling caused by an abnormal accumulation of fluid is called:

A. edema
B. emesis
C. hemostasis
D. hematoma

235. If a phlebotomist notes that the arm selected for venipuncture is edematous, he or she should:

A. perform the venipuncture
B. notify the patient's nurse
C. select another site
D. write "Can't get" on the requisition

236. Which of the following conditions occuring in edematous tissues may alter test results?

A. destruction of platelets
B. destruction of red blood cells
C. dislodging of the platelet plug
D. injury of fragile tissue

237. Which of the following veins is often the most accessible in obese patients?

A. basilic vein
B. cephalic vein
C. median cubital vein
D. median vein of the forearm

238. Veins that are hardened are:

A. elastic
B. resilient
C. sclerosed
D. spongy

239. If a phlebotomist palpates a vein and determines that it is sclerosed, the phlebotomist should:

A. draw above the sclerosed area
B. draw below the sclerosed area
C. notify the patient's physician
D. turn off the IV and perform the draw

240. Which of the following is a cause of sclerosed veins?

A. numerous venipunctures
B. radical mastectomy
C. residual alcohol
C. residual iodine

241. If a phlebotomist must collect a blood specimen from a patient's arm that has an IV, the phlebotomist should draw from:

A. above the IV
B. below the IV
C. the IV line directly
D. the patient's CVC

242. During routine venipuncture, after the phlebotomist engages the evacuated tube, no blood appears in the tube. The phlebotomist determines that the venipuncture attempt was unsuccessful. What should the phlebotomist do FIRST to end the procedure?

A. call the nurse
B. tighten the tourniquet
C. untie the tourniquet
D. withdraw the needle

243. During venipuncture, the phlebotomist inserts the needle next to the patient's vein, on the left side of the patient's vein. No blood appears in the evacuated tube. The phlebotomist should:

A. completely withdraw the needle
B. insert the needle deeper
C. pull back and reinsert the needle to the left
D. pull back and reinsert the needle to the right

244. The following colored tubes with conventional stoppers are to be collected during routine venipuncture: red SST, yellow (SPS), sky blue, green. According to NCCLS guidelines, in what sequence should the tubes be collected, following venipuncture?

A. red SST, yellow, sky blue, green
B. red SST, sky blue, green, yellow
C. yellow, red SST, sky blue, green
D. yellow, red SST, green, sky blue

245. The following colored tubes with conventional stoppers are to be collected during routine venipuncture: gray, red, blue, lavender. Accoring to NCCLS guidelines, in what sequence should the tubes be collected, following venipuncture?

A. blue, gray, lavender, red
B. gray, blue, lavender, red
C. red, blue, lavender, gray
D. red, gray, blue, lavender

246. The following colored tubes with conventional stoppers are to be collected during routine venipuncture: red SST, lavender, gray, sky blue. According to NCCLS guidelines, which tube stopper color should be collected *first,* following venipuncture?

A. gray
B. lavender
C. red SST
D. sky blue

247. The following colored tubes with conventional stoppers are to be collected during routine venipuncture: green, gray, lavender, black. According to NCCLS guidelines, which evacuated tube stopper color should be collected *first?*

A. black
B. green
C. gray
D. lavender

248. The following colored tubes with conventional stoppers are to be collected during routine venipuncture: lavender, red SST, sky blue, yellow (containing SPS). According to NCCLS guidelines, which tube stopper color should be collected *first?*

A. lavender
B. red SST
C. sky blue
D. yellow

249. The following colored tubes with conventional stoppers are to be collected during routine venipuncture: lavender, red SST, sky blue, yellow (SPS). According to NCCLS guidelines, which tube should be collected *last?*

A. lavender
B. red SST
C. sky blue
D. yellow

250. The following colored tubes with conventional stoppers are to be collected during routine venipuncture: green, gray, red SST, sky blue. According to NCCLS guidelines, which tube should be collected *last?*

A. green
B. gray
C. red SST
D. sky blue

251. A phlebotomist is to collect a specimen for an APTT and prothrombin time from a patient. According to NCCLS guidelines, what tube stopper color should the phlebotomist collect *first?*

A. green
B. gray
C. red
D. sky blue

252. The following colored tubes with Hemogard™ stoppers are to be collected during routine venipuncture: gold, green, gray, lavender. According to NCCLS guidelines, which tube should be collected *first?*

A. gold
B. green
C. gray
D. lavender

253. The rationale for the sequence of multiple specimen collection following venipuncture is to prevent:

A. contamination
B. glycolysis
C. hemolysis
D. platelet clumping

254. The condition characterized by deep and rapid respiration preceding the onset of muscular twitching and contractions is called:

A. hematoma
B. hemolysis
C. syncope
D. tetany

255. The condition characterized by dizziness, weakness, pallor, clammy skin, and unconsciousness is called:

A. hematoma
B. hemolysis
C. syncope
D. tetany

256. The condition characterized by a purple area surrounding a venipuncture site, accompanied by swelling, is called:

A. hematoma
B. hemolysis
C. syncope
D. tetany

257. The condition characterized by small reddish-purple spots on a patient's skin is called:

A. hematoma
B. hemolysis
C. petechiae
D. syncope

258. The term that describes the backward flow of blood into a patient's veins during venipuncture is:

A. hematoma
B. hemolysis
C. reflux
D. rouleaux

259. What response may some patients have at the sight of their blood being drawn?

A. hematoma
B. hemolysis
C. syncope
D. synergy

260. Which of the following conditions may be caused by a needle penetrating all the way through the vein during venipuncture?

A. hematoma
B. hemolysis
C. syncope
D. synergy

261. Which of the following may cause petechiae on a patient's skin?

A. allergy to the iodine
B. blood leaking into the tissues
C. patient platelet defects
D. the sight of blood

262. During venipuncture, a phlebotomist moves the tube gently up and down in the holder, moving the contents back and forth. What may this cause?

A. hematoma
B. hemolysis
C. petechiae
D. reflux

263. The condition in which the plasma portion of the blood filters into the tissues is called:

A. hematoma
B. hemoconcentration
C. hemolysis
D. hemostasis

264. Hemoconcentration of the specimen may be caused by:

A. drawing from a hematoma
B. prolonged tourniquet application
C. residual alcohol on the site
D. shaking an additive tube

265. Hemoconcentration of the specimen may be caused by:

A. drawing from a hematoma
B. residual alcohol on the site
C. shaking additive tubes
D. vigorous hand pumping

266. Using a needle that is too small to accommodate the force of the vacuum of an evacuated tube may cause which of the following in a patient's specimen?

A. hemoconcentration
B. hemolysis
C. hemostasis
D. hematoma

267. Shaking an evacuated tube containing an additive too forcefully to mix the contents may cause which of the following in a patient's specimen?

A. hemoconcentration
B. hemolysis
C. hemostasis
D. hematoma

268. Drawing blood through a hematoma may cause which of the following in a patient's specimen?

A. hemoconcentration
B. hemolysis
C. hemostasis
D. hematoma

269. Obtaining a specimen as a result of a traumatic venipuncture can cause which of the following in a patient's specimen?

A. hemoconcentration
B. hemolysis
C. hemostasis
D. hematoma

270. A patient suffers a transfusion reaction. What may this condition cause in the patient's specimen?

A. hemoconcentration
B. hemolysis
C. hemostasis
D. hematoma

271. If a specimen is hemolyzed, what color is the serum?

A. green
B. pink
C. white
D. yellow

272. Which of the following analyses requires an arterial specimen?

A. blood alcohol levels
B. blood culture
C. blood gas analysis
D. blood urea nitrogen

273. Which of the following departments in the health care setting relies most heavily on ABG results?

A. occupational therapy
B. physical therapy
C. radiation therapy
D. respiratory therapy

274. Involuntary contraction of an artery is called:

A. agglutination
B. arrhythmia
C. arteriosclerosis
D. arteriospasm

275. A process where blood is provided to a part of the body by more than one blood vessel is called:

A. Allen test
B. iontophoresis
C. collapsed vein
D. collateral circulation

276. Which of the following structures is located on the lateral aspect of the wrist?

A. radial artery
B. ulnar artery
C. deep palmar arch
D. superficial palmar arch

277. Which of the following structures is located on the medial aspect of the wrist?

A. brachial artery
B. femoral artery
C. radial artery
D. ulnar artery

278. Which of the following structures is located in the leg?

A. brachial artery
B. femoral artery
C. radial artery
D. ulnar artery

279. Which of the following structures is located in the medial anterior aspect of the antecubital fossa?

A. brachial artery
B. femoral artery
C. radial artery
D. ulnar artery

280. Which of the following tests is performed to assess collateral circulation of a patient's hand prior to arterial puncture?

A. Allen test
B. mucin clot test
C. Ropes test
D. sweat chloride test

281. Listed below are several sites commonly used for arterial puncture. Which site offers the advantage of collateral circulation?

A. brachial artery
B. femoral artery
C. radial artery
D. ulnar artery

282. Listed below are several sites commonly used for arterial puncture. Which is the second choice for arterial puncture?

A. brachial artery
B. femoral artery
C. radial artery
D. ulnar artery

283. Listed below are several sites commonly used for arterial puncture. Which site offers the advantage of largest size?

A. brachial artery
B. femoral artery
C. radial artery
D. ulnar artery

284. Listed below are several sites commonly used for arterial puncture. Which site has the disadvantage of being located close to the basilic vein?

A. brachial artery
B. femoral artery
C. radial artery
D. ulnar artery

285. Listed below are several sites commonly used for arterial puncture. Which site has the disadvantage of increased risk of infection?

A. brachial artery
B. femoral artery
C. radial artery
D. ulnar artery

286. During the Allen test, which two arteries are compressed by the phlebotomist?

A. brachial and femoral
B. brachial and radial
C. femoral and radial
D. radial and ulnar

287. During the Allen test, which artery is released FIRST?

A. brachial
B. femoral
C. radial
D. ulnar

288. During the Allen test, two arteries are compressed. One artery is subsequently released. If normal circulation is present, the patient's hand should turn pink within how many seconds?

A. 5
B. 7
C. 9
D. 10

289. During an Allen test, a patient's hand returns to pink 10 seconds after one of the arteries is released. What should the phlebotomist do next?

A. call a code
B. perform Allen test on another site
C. select the brachial artery for arterial puncture
D. select the artery tested for arterial puncture

290. Which of the following supplies would a phlebotomist carry on his or her tray to collect samples for ABG analysis?

A. alcohol, tourniquet, syringe
B. alcohol, syringe, rubber stopper
C. iodine, syringe, aluminum foil
D. alcohol, iodine, tourniquet

291. Which of the following blood vessel characteristics is helpful to a phlebotomist, when palpating for a suitable site for arterial puncture?

A. pulse
B. elastic structure
C. ropelike structure
D. spongy texture

292. Which of the following equipment is used routinely for venipuncture, but not arterial puncture?

A. alcohol
B. iodine
C. warmer
D. tourniquet

293. Which of the following anticoagulants is used for the collection of specimens for ABG analysis?

A. EDTA
B. SPS
C. heparin
D. oxalate

294. The phlebotomist should inform a patient that the ABG procedure is:

A. less painful, compared venipuncture
B. more painful, compared venipuncture
C. as painful as venipuncture
D. a painless procedure

295. Which of the following equipment is used to collect specimens for ABG analysis?

A. evacuated tube
B. Microtainer™
C. syringe
D. Unopette™

296. At what angle should the needle be inserted during an arterial puncture procedure?

A. 15 degrees
B. 30 degrees
C. 45 degrees
D. 60 degrees

297. Which of the following tests requires that the puncture site be warmed prior to collection?

A. capillary blood gas analysis
B. PKU analysis
C. sickle cell screen
D. T3, T4 analysis

298. Which of the following is used to mix the specimen with the collection tube additive during capillary blood gas specimen collection?

A. agitator
B. clay
C. metal flea
D. rotator

299. Following collection, how should specimens collected for ABGs be transported?

A. at 37°C
B. on ice
C. routinely
D. shielded from light

300. A phlebotomist collected a specimen for ABG analysis. What should the phlebotomist do with the needle, after withdrawing it from the patient's arm?

A. insert it into a cork stopper
B. insert it into a rubber stopper
C. place it in a biohazard bag
D. place it in a sharps container

301. Which of the following complications may occur following arterial puncture, but not venipuncture?

A. arteriospasm
B. hematoma
C. infection
D. thrombus formation

302. A sudden, transient constriction of an artery in response to pain or other stimuli is called:

A. arteriospasm
B. hematoma
C. reflux
D. thrombus

303. Pressure is applied to an arterial puncture site for at least 5 minutes following a procedure to prevent:

A. arteriospasm
B. hematoma
C. reflux
D. thrombus formation

304. A physician would most likely order a blood culture on a patient who has:

A. AGL
B. CAB
C. FUO
D. UCHD

305. Which of the following concerns is important when collecting specimens for blood culture analysis?

A. preventing air bubbles in the specimen
B. using heparin
C. using sterile technique to prepare the site
D. transporting the specimen on ice

306. The presence of bacteria and their toxins in the bloodstream is called:

A. bacteremia
B. basophilia
C. hyperemia
D. septicemia

307. The term that means "without air" is:

A. aerobic
B. anaerobic
C. afebrile
D. antimicrobial

308. A phlebotomist must collect a specimen for a blood culture analysis. The phlebotomist should prepare the venipuncture site using:

A. alcohol only
B. iodine only
C. alcohol and iodine
D. tincture of green soap

309. Contamination rates of blood culture specimens should not exceed:

A. 0%
B. 3%
C. 6%
D. 10%

310. Which of the following actions may result in a false positive blood culture result?

A. collecting blood in an SPS evacuated tube
B. introducing iodine into the collection container
C. leaving the tourniquet on too long
D. repalpating the site

311. Which of the following tests may require an extra step in patient identification?

A. blood cultures
B. cold agglutinin titers
C. glucose tolerance testing
D. type and crossmatch

312. Which of the following blood collection techniques requires sterile technique to prepare a venipuncture site?

A. blood culture
B. cold agglutinin titers
C. glucose tolerance testing
D. type and crossmatch

313. Which of the following specimens requires warming a collection tube to 37°C?

A. blood culture
B. cold agglutinin titers
C. glucose tolerance testing
D. type and screen

314. Which of the following procedures requires a patient to refrain from strenuous exercise for 12 hours prior to the test?

A. blood culture
B. cold agglutinin titer
C. glucose tolerance test
D. type and screen

315. Which of the following tests requires that a patient fast prior to collection of the blood specimen?

A. blood culture
B. cold agglutinin titer
C. glucose tolerance testing
D. type and crossmatch

316. Introducing bacteria from a patient's skin into a specimen for blood culture analysis may result in:

A. false negative results
B. false positive results
C. hemoconcentration
D. hemolysis

317. Introducing iodine into a specimen for blood culture analysis can result in:

A. false negative results
B. false positive results
C. hemoconcentration
D. hemolysis

318. Repalpating a site prior to venipuncture for blood culture analysis, may result in:

A. false negative results
B. false positive results
C. hemoconcentration
D. hemolysis

319. Introducing air into an anaerobic blood culture collection container may result in:

A. false negative results
B. false positive results
C. hemoconcentration
D. hemolysis

320. Which of the following conventional stopper colors corresponds to the evacuated tube suitable for blood culture specimen collection?

A. lavender
B. royal blue
C. sky blue
D. yellow

321. Which of the following evacuated tube additives inhibits complement?

A. sodium citrate
B. sodium heparin
C. EDTA
D. SPS

322. Which of the following tests would be most affected by lack of proper patient preparation?

A. blood cultures
B. fibrin degradation products
C. glucose tolerance testing
D. type and crossmatch

323. Which of the following blood culture specimen collection containers incorporates an aerobic bottle and an anaerobic bottle?

A. Bactec™ system
B. gas impermeable syringe
C. SPS evacuated tube/conventional stopper
D. SPS evacuated tube/Hemogard™ closure

324. While performing a venipuncture with a syringe, a phlebotomist notices blood frothing between the hub of the needle and the syringe. As a result, the specimen may be:

A. activated
B. contaminated
C. hemolyzed
D. iontophoresced

325. A specimen collected by syringe is hemolyzed. What may have caused this?

A. aliquoting specimens in the wrong order
B. forcefully drawing back the plunger
C. gently drawing back the plunger
D. gently inverting the specimen tubes

326. Following venipuncture by syringe, blood must be aliquoted into the following evacuated tubes: red, sky blue, green. In what order should the evacuated tubes be filled?

A. green, red, sky blue
B. red, green, sky blue
C. red, sky blue, green
D. sky blue, green, red

327. The rationale for the order of draw for syringes is to minimize:

A. cross contamination of specimens
B. clotting in anticoagulant tubes
C. hemolysis of the specimen
D. platelet clumping

328. Which of the following is increased, compared with the antecubital fossa, on the skin surface of the hand?

A. bacteria
B. endothelial casts
C. number of arteries
D. number of veins

329. Which step in the venipuncture procedure must the phlebotomist exercise extra care in performing when collecting blood by venipuncture from a hand vein?

A. anchoring the vein
B. labeling the specimen
C. needle insertion
D. tourniquet application

330. Why is the fifth finger of a patient's hand routinely eliminated as a potential site for skin puncture?

A. it has a pulse
B. it has an increased number of nerve endings
C. the tissue is thinner than other fingers
D. it is usually calloused

331. Why is the index finger of a patient's hand routinely eliminated as a potential site for skin puncture?

A. it has a pulse
B. it has an increased number of nerve endings
C. the tissue is thinner than other fingers
D. it is usually calloused

332. Which of the following blood constituents may be falsely elevated if the skin puncture site is prepared with povidone iodine?

A. hemoglobin
B. hepatitis B surface antigen
C. platelet count
D. potassium

333. Which of the following constituents is present in higher concentrations in blood collected by skin puncture than in blood collected by venipuncture?

A. calcium
B. glucose
C. potassium
D. total protein

334. Which of the following skin puncture specimens is most likely to be adversely affected by excessive squeezing of the site?

A. bedside glucose test from a 75-year-old woman
B. bilirubin test from a 12-hour-old neonate
C. microhematocrit determination from a 30-year-old donor
D. WBC and platelet count from a 65-year-old oncology patient

335. Positioning a patient's arm downward prior to venipuncture will help prevent:

A. hemoconcentration
B. hemolysis
C. reflux
D. syncope

336. A phlebotomist attempts a venipuncture on a patient's basilic vein. If the blood that appears in the evacuated tube is dark purple-red, the phlebotomist should:

A. allow the tube to fill, following standard procedures
B. immediately release the tourniquet and withdraw the needle
C. insert the needle deeper
D. withdraw the needle, and apply pressure for 5 minutes

337. A phlebotomist selects a 4.5 mL sodium citrate tube to collect a patient's specimen. The patient was difficult to draw, but the phlebotomist successfully collected approximately 3.0 mL of specimen into the sodium citrate tube. The phlebotomist should next

A. gently invert the specimen 5 to 10 times
B. label the specimen
C. recollect the specimen
D. shield the specimen from light

338. If a patient's arms and hands are swollen due to excessive fluid retention, this patient's condition is called:

A. edema
B. hemolysis
C. petechiae
D. syncope

339. A specimen for ABG analysis would be rejected if the specimen:

A. contained air bubbles
B. included the needle attached to the syringe
C. was collected in heparin
D. was transported on ice

340. Clinically significant changes will occur in a specimen collected for ABG analysis if the specimen is left at room temperature for more than:

A. 5 to 10 minutes
B. 10 to 15 minutes
C. 15 to 20 minutes
D. 20 to 25 minutes

341. A phlebotomist attempts an arterial puncture of the brachial artery. If the blood appearing in the syringe is bright orange-red, the phlebotomist should:

A. apply an ice pack
B. call a code
C. continue the procedure
D. discontinue the procedure

342. Which of the following situations will be caused if too much heparin is in the syringe used to collect a specimen for ABG analysis?

A. acidosis of the specimen
B. alkalosis of the specimen
C. excessive bleeding
D. hematoma formation

343. A syringe used for collection of ABG samples should be:

A. blue
B. green
C. gas impermeable
D. gas permeable

344. What is the maximum number of venipuncture attempts a phlebotomist should make to secure a specimen?

A. 1
B. 2
C. 3
D. 4

345. What is the maximum length of time that a tourniquet may be left on a patient's arm without adversely affecting test results?

A. 1 minute
B. 3 minutes
C. 5 minutes
D. 7 minutes

346. Which of the following evacuated tubes must always be preceded by a discard tube?

A. green
B. lavender
C. red SST
D. sky blue

347. What is the maximum number of times a phlebotomist should perform skin puncture on an infant's foot to secure a specimen?

A. 1
B. 2
C. 3
D. 4

CHAPTER 3

Specimen Processing and Handling

348. Listed below are colors of conventional stoppers for evacuated tubes. Which stopper color would be selected most often to collect specimens analyzed in the chemistry department?

    A. green
    B. gray
    C. lavender
    D. red SST

349. Listed below are colors of conventional stoppers for evacuated tubes. Which stopper color would be selected most often to collect specimens analyzed by the hematology department?

    A. gray
    B. lavender
    C. light blue
    D. red SST

350. Which of the following departments in the clinical laboratory performs ASO titers, cold agglutinin titers, and rapid plasma reagin analyses?

    A. clinical chemistry
    B. hematology
    C. immunology
    D. microbiology

351. Which of the following laboratory departments offers a profile of tests that analyzes amylase, bilirubin, electrolytes, glucose, ALT, AST, BUN, and LDH?

    A. clinical chemistry
    B. hematology
    C. immunology
    D. microbiology

352. Which of the following departments in the clinical laboratory is most often responsible for analyzing specimens for prothrombin time and APTT analysis?

A. clinical chemistry
B. coagulation
C. immunology
D. microbiology

353. Which department of the clinical laboratory is most likely to perform an AFB culture?

A. clinical chemistry
B. hematology
C. immunology
D. microbiology

354. Which of the following colored conventional stoppers for evacuated tubes would most likely be delivered to microbiology for analysis?

A. lavender
B. light blue
C. red SST
D. yellow

355. Which of the following departments would most likely perform a type and crossmatch analysis?

A. clinical chemistry
B. hematology
C. immunology
D. immunohematology

356. Listed below are colors of conventional stoppers for evacuated tubes. Which stopper color would be selected most often to collect specimens analyzed in the immunohematology department?

A. red
B. red SST
C. light blue
D. royal blue

357. The condition when the patient is at rest, in a supine position, 12 hours after the last ingestion of food, exercise, or activity is:

A. basal state
B. diurnal rhythms
C. normal
D. reference value

358. Normal variations of blood constituents throughout the day are called:

A. basal state
B. diurnal rhythms
C. normal
D. reference value

359. Normal spans of values for laboratory tests are called:

A. basal state
B. diurnal rhythms
C. normal
D. reference value

360. A clinical situation in which the water from the plasma portion of the blood filters into the tissues, causing nonfilterable values in the blood to falsely increase, is called:

A. hemoconcentration
B. hemolysis
C. hematology
D. hematoma

361. Cloudy serum or plasma caused by an increased lipid content is called:

A. diurnal rhythms
B. hemoconcentration
C. hemolysis
D. lipemic

362. If a patient finishes drinking a glucose solution during a GTT at 7:30 AM, what time should the first specimen be drawn?

A. 7:45 AM
B. 8:00 AM
C. 8:15 AM
D. 8:30 AM

363. Which of the following tests is usually ordered as a series of samples collected at timed intervals?

A. blood cultures
B. cold agglutinin titers
C. cryoglobulin levels
D. fibrin degradation products

364. If a physician orders a 3-hour glucose tolerance test on a patient, how many blood collection procedures must be performed as part of the GTT?

A. 2
B. 3
C. 4
D. 5

365. When labeling blood culture specimens, what information is required in addition to routine labeling information?

A. patient's age
B. patient's gender
C. number of the series
D. number of venipuncture attempts

366. When labeling a blood culture specimen, what information should a phlebotomist record, in addition to routine labeling information?

A. time of last venipuncture
B. date of last venipuncture
C. nurse's initials
D. venipuncture site used

367. At what temperature do cold agglutinins react best?

A. 4°C
B. 23°C
C. 37°C
D. 56°C

368. Collection of blood specimens for which of the following tests may incorporate the use of a Typenex™ band?

A. blood cultures
B. glucose tolerance testing
C. fibrin split products
D. type and crossmatch

369. Which of the following would appear in addition to routine labeling information on a specimen collected as part of a GTT?

A. skin puncture site selected
B. timing of the specimen
C. Typenex™ numbers
D. venipuncture site selected

370. Which of the following specimens requires transport shielded from light?

A. alkaline phosphatase
B. bilirubin
C. cold agglutinin
D. fibrinogen

371. Which of the following specimens requires transport shielded from light?

A. acid phosphatase
B. blood urea nitrogen
C. carotene
D. fibrin split products

372. Which of the following specimens requires transport shielded from light?

A. ammonia
B. electrolytes
C. erythrocyte protoporphyrin level
D. gastrin

373. Which of the following specimens must be transported at 37°C?

A. carotene
B. catecholamines
C. cold agglutinin titers
D. creatine phosphokinase

374. Which of the following materials is most commonly used to transport specimens shielded from light?

A. aluminum foil
B. paper cup
C. paper towel
D. plastic bag

375. Specimens that must be transported chilled should be transported:

A. on dry ice
B. in a cup filled with ice cubes
C. in a cup filled with ice cubes and water
D. wrapped in a cold pack

376. What is the best method for transporting specimens at 37°C?

A. ice bath
B. heat block
C. wrapped in a towel
D. wrapped in a washcloth dampened with warm water

377. Which of the following specimens requires chilled transport?

A. albumin
B. ammonia
C. amylase
D. antibody screen

378. Which of the following specimens requires chilled transport?

A. febrile agglutinins
B. folate
C. fibrinogen
D. follicle stimulating hormone

379. Which of the following specimens requires chilled transport?

A. gastrin
B. gentamycin
C. glucose
D. glucose-6-phosphate dehydrogenase

380. Which of the following specimens requires chilled transport?

A. rapid plasma reagin
B. renin
C. reticulocyte count
D. RhoGAM workup

381. If a laboratory test procedure requested by a physician cannot be analyzed by the in-house laboratory, the specimen should be sent to which type of laboratory?

A. point of care
B. reference
C. satellite
D. stat

382. Which of the following containers should hold a specimen that has been wrapped in absorbent material for transport to a reference lab?

A. gas impermeable container
B. primary container
C. secondary container
D. shipping container

383. Which of the following characteristics applies to a drug that is monitored by a therapeutic drug monitoring system?

A. administered IV only
B. administered "stat"
C. narrow therapeutic-toxic ranges
D. predicable dose-response relationships

384. Which of the following drugs is characteristically incorporated into a TDM program?

A. acetaminophen
B. aminoglycosides
C. morphine
D. salicylate

385. Which of the following is a common reason for rejection of specimens collected as part of a TDM program?

A. failure to collect specimen at the appropriate time
B. failure to mix blood with additive
C. incorrect specimen tube
D. insufficient specimen

386. Before a specimen for TDM can be collected, there must be verification of the patient's last:

A. meal
B. medication dose
C. therapy session
D. venipuncture

387. A TDM specimen that is collected approximately 30 minutes prior to the next scheduled dose is for what type of medication level?

A. peak
B. random
C. toxic
D. trough

388. A phlebotomist is to collect a blood specimen at 7:00 AM as part of a TDM program. The phlebotomist has several specimens to collect at that time. How many minutes before or after the hour can she or he collect the specimen?

A. 0
B. 5
C. 10
D. 15

389. What kind of form must be completed for forensic specimens?

A. chain of custody
B. chordae tendineae
C. incident report
D. respondeat superior

390. Which of the following agencies defines requirements for the collection, processing, and testing of urine drug screens?

A. ASCP
B. ASMT
C. NCCLS
D. NIDA

391. Which of the following security measures is routinely performed by collection sites for urine drug testing to ensure specimen integrity?

A. accept catheterized specimens only
B. collect in a sterile container
C. collect using a Simplate™
D. place bluing material in the toilet

392. What is the minimum acceptable volume of a specimen for urine drug screening, according to NIDA?

A. 30 mL
B. 40 mL
C. 50 mL
D. 60 mL

393. What temperature range must a urine specimen fall within to be accepted for drug screening, according to NIDA guidelines?

A. 90.5 to 95.5°F
B. 95.5 to 99.8°F
C. 90.5 to 99.8°F
D. 98.6 to 99°F

394. Which of the following laboratory tests may be performed on a random urine specimen?

A. 2 hour urine collection
B. 24 hour urine collection
C. urinalysis
D. urine culture and sensitivity

395. Which of the following laboratory tests requires a clean-catch midstream urine collection?

A. 2 hour urine collection
B. 24 hour urine collection
C. urinalysis
D. urine culture and sensitivity

396. Following collection, a specimen for urine culture and sensitivity must be delivered to the laboratory:

A. within 60 minutes
B. within 90 minutes
C. within 120 minutes
D. stat

397. If a urine specimen cannot be delivered to the laboratory immediately following collection, the specimen should be stored:

A. at room temperature
B. in a 37°C incubator
C. in a refrigerator
D. shielded from the light

398. A specimen for routine urinalysis must be delivered to the laboratory following collection within:

A. 60 minutes
B. 90 minutes
C. 120 minutes
D. 180 minutes

399. If a phlebotomist uses a sterile cotton swab to brush a patient's tonsillar area and the posterior pharynx, what specimen has the phlebotomist collected?

A. ascitic fluid
B. nasopharyngeal culture
C. synovial fluid
D. throat culture

400. Arterial blood gas specimens require special transport to prevent changes in:

A. bilirubin levels
B. carotene levels
C. glucose levels
D. pH levels

401. Which of the following analyses is always transported and analyzed stat?

A. ABG
B. BUN
C. CBC
D. RPR

402. The term that means "immediately" is:

A. ASAP
B. FYI
C. med emerg
D stat

403. Blood specimens from which patient unit are always handled as stat requests?

A. ER
B. ICU
C. labor and delivery
D. pediatrics

404. Which of the following analyses requires the patient to fast prior to collection?

A. C-reactive protein
B. creatine phosphokinase
C. creatinine
D. cytomegalovirus

405. Which of the following analyses requires the patient to fast prior to collection?

A. plasma hemoglobin
B. hemoglobin A1C
C. renin
D. serum gastrin

406. Which of the following analyses requires the patient to fast prior to collection?

A. theophylline
B. thrombin time
C. tobramycin
D. triglycerides

407. The department in the clinical laboratory that identifies disease of blood-forming tissues is:

A. clinical chemistry
B. hematology
C. immunology
D. microbiology

408. The department in the clinical laboratory, often housed in the hematology department, that monitors medication given as anticoagulant therapy is:

A. clinical chemistry
B. coagulation
C. microbiology
D. urinalysis

409. The department in the clinical laboratory that cultures and identifies bacterial pathogens is:

A. clinical chemistry
B. hematology
C. microbiology
D. urinalysis

410. The department in the clinical laboratory that analyzes antibody-antigen reactions prior to the transfusion of blood or blood products is:

A. clinical chemistry
B. immunohematology
C. immunology
D. radioimmunoassay

411. The department in the clinical laboratory that assesses the body's response to certain infectious diseases through the analysis of antigen-antibody reactions is:

A. clinical chemistry
B. hematology
C. immunohematology
D. immunology

412. The department of the clinical laboratory that conducts testing of the antibodies and antigens associated with hepatitis, and certain hormone and drug levels is:

A. clinical chemistry
B. immunology
C. microbiology
D. radioimmunoassay

413. The department in the clinical laboratory that screens for the early detection of cancer cells is:

A. clinical microscopy
B. cytology
C. hematology
D. histology

414. The department in the clinical laboratory that prepares and processes tissue samples removed during surgery is:

A. clinical microscopy
B. cytology
C. hematology
D. histology

415. A test commonly ordered to assist in the diagnosis of cystic fibrosis is:

A. mucin clot test
B. Ropes test
C. sweat chloride test
D. tourniquet test

416. A patient has a chloride level in his or her sweat that is five times the normal level. What clinical condition is most often associated with this finding?

A. cystic fibrosis
B. hyaline membrane disease
C. PKU
D. PNI

417. The process of introducing ions into the skin through the use of electrodes placed on the skin is called:

A. electrophoresis
B. iontophoresis
C. leukopheresis
D. plasmapheresis

418. To accept a specimen for trace metal analysis, the specimen should be collected in a(an):

A. acid-washed plastic syringe
B. gas impermeable syringe
C. red stopper evacuated tube
D. red SST stopper evacuated tube

419. Listed below are colors of Hemogard™ stoppers for evacuated tubes. Which Hemogard™ stoppered evacuated tube is most suitable for lead level determinations?

A. brown
B. gold
C. gray
D. red

420. Listed below are colors of hemogard stoppers for evacuated tubes. Which Hemogard™ stoppered evacuated tube is most suitable for zinc level determinations?

A. brown
B. gold
C. light blue
D. royal blue

421. To accept a specimen for fibrin split product analysis, the specimen should be collected in a(an):

A. acid washed syringe
B. gas impermeable syringe
C. royal blue Hemogard™ stoppered tube
D. Thrombo-Wellcotest™ tube

422. Which of the following test procedures is preceded by a GTT?

A. glucagon tolerance test
B. lactose tolerance test
C. sweat chloride test
D. D-xylose test

423. According to NCCLS, what is the maximum time that may elapse between collection of a blood specimen and separation of the cells from the sera?

A. 30 minutes
B. 45 minutes
C. 1 hour
D. 2 hours

424. Which of the following test results will be affected by glycolytic action of the red blood cells?

A. CBC
B. WBC
C. glucose
D. vancomycin

425. A specimen for glucose analysis is collected in an evacuated tube with a red stopper. The specimen was not processed in a timely fashion. As a result, the serum glucose values:

A. decreased
B. increased
C. were impossible to analyze
D. were unaffected

426. A specimen for glucose analysis is collected in a red stoppered SST evacuated tube. The specimen was centrifuged promptly, but not analyzed in a timely fashion. As a result, the serum glucose values:

A. decreased
B. increased
C. were impossible to analyze
D. were unaffected

427. A specimen for potassium analysis is collected in an evacuated tube with a red stopper. The specimen was centrifuged promptly, but not analyzed in a timely fashion. As a result, the serum potassium values:

A. decreased
B. increased
C. were impossible to analyze
D. were unaffected

428. A specimen for potassium analysis is collected in a red stoppered SST evacuated tube. The specimen was centrifuged promptly, but not analyzed in a timely fashion. As a result, the serum potassium values:

A. decreased
B. increased
C. were impossible to analyze
D. were unaffected

429. What advantage does a pneumatic tube delivery system offer?

A. decreases specimen delivery time
B. increases specimen delivery time
C. reduces contamination risks to personnel
D. reduces the number of hemolyzed blood specimens

430. If a specimen is left uncovered, which of the following test results may be affected?

A. alcohol
B. potassium
C. type and crossmatch
D. type and screen

431. If the specimen is contaminated with talc, which of the following test results may be affected?

A. CBC
B. WBC
C. calcium
D. potassium

432. Neonatal specimens for PKU analysis should be collected using:

A. filter paper
B. glass slides
C. Microtainer™ tubes
D. Unopette™ system

433. Following collection, filter paper specimens should be dried at which of the following temperatures?

A. 4°C
B. 20°C
C. 37°C
D. 56°C

434. Following collection, filter paper specimens should be dried horizontally for at least how long?

A. 1 hour
B. 2 hours
C. 3 hours
D. 4 hours

435. At what angle should filter paper specimens be stacked, prior to transport to the laboratory that will perform the analysis?

A. 15
B. 45
C. 90
D. 180

436. Which of the following collection devices is used to transfer neonatal capillary specimens to filter paper?

A. heparinized capillary tubes
B. plain capillary tubes
C. MLA™ pipette
D. Unopette™ pipette

437. Within how many hours must filter paper specimens be mailed to the laboratory following collections?

A. 3 hours
B. 6 hours
C. 24 hours
D. 48 hours

438. What type of measurement system is most often used in bedside glucose testing analyzers?

A. refractometer
B. reflectometer
C. tachometer
D. T/S meter

439. Which of the following terms refers to obtaining a part of a patient's specimen for analysis?

A. accession
B. aliquot
C. centrifuge
D. filter

440. At what speed are most blood specimens usually centrifuged?

A. 250 to 500g
B. 500 to 750g
C. 850 to 1000g
D. 1000 to 2000g

441. A phlebotomist has placed several blood specimens into the centrifuge and started it. If the centrifuge begins to vibrate, the phlebotomist should:

A. call a code
B. call the security department
C. pull the fire alarm
D. turn off the centrifuge

442. If blood specimens have been placed in a centrifuge correctly, they will be placed:

A. at random in the centrifuge
B. on the left side of the centrifuge
C. on the right side of the centrifuge
D. similar sized tubes opposite each other

443. To safely remove stoppers from evacuated tubes, the phlebotomist should use:

A. an alcohol prep pad
B. a centrifuge
C. gauze
D. a pipette

444. How long following collection must a phlebotomist wait for a specimen collected in a red stoppered SST evacuated tube to clot?

A. 0 minutes
B. 15 minutes
C. 30 minutes
D. 60 minutes

445. How long following collection must a phlebotomist wait to centrifuge a specimen collected in a green stoppered PST evacuated tube?

A. 0 minutes
B. 15 minutes
C. 30 minutes
D. 60 minutes

446. If the serum of a specimen collected for type and crossmatch is hemolyzed, the medical laboratory technician should:

A. perform the type and crossmatch
B. perform a type and screen only
C. refer the specimen to a reference lab
D. reject the specimen

447. If a specimen collected for cold agglutinin analysis was collected in a gel separation tube, the MLT should:

A. accept the specimen
B. reject the specimen
C. warm the specimen
D. send the specimen to a reference lab

448. A patient's requisition form reads, "Jane Jones." If the label on the corresponding specimen reads, "J. Jones," the MLT should:

A. ask the PBT to use full names on all future labels and analyze
B. accept the specimen
C. change the label
D. reject the specimen

449. Listed below are colors of conventional stoppers for evacuated tubes. Which stopper color would be selected most often to collect specimens analyzed in the coagulation department?

A. green
B. red
C. light blue
D. royal blue

450. Listed below are colors of conventional stoppers for evacuated tubes. Which stopper color would be selected most often to collect specimens analyzed in the hematology department?

A. green
B. lavender
C. light blue
D. royal blue

CHAPTER 4

Laboratory Operations

451. The government agency of the United States responsible for regulating the safety and health of workers is:

 A. ASCP
 B. CAP
 C. JCAHO
 D. OSHA

452. The agency that developed a label designed to communicate specific hazards associated with hazardous chemicals is:

 A. ASCP
 B. CAP
 C. JCAHO
 D. NFPA

453. According to the National Fire Protection Agency, which of the following classes of fires occurs with ordinary combustibles?

 A. A
 B. B
 C. C
 D. D

454. According to the National Fire Protection Agency, which of the following classes of fires occurs with flammable liquids and vapors?

 A. A
 B. B
 C. C
 D. D

455. According to the National Fire Protection Agency, which of the following classes of fires occurs with electrical equipment?

A. A
B. B
C. C
D. D

456. According to the National Fire Protection Agency, which of the following classes of fires occurs with combustible or reactive metals?

A. A
B. B
C. C
D. D

457. What is the National Fire Protection Agency's code word for action in the event of a fire?

A. EDTA
B. OSHA
C. PASS
D. RACE

458. Which of the following mnemonics communicates the appropriate procedure to follow when using a fire extinguisher?

A. EDTA
B. OSHA
C. PASS
D. RACE

459. Which of the following fire extinguisher contents is appropriate to use on a Class A fire?

A. carbon dioxide
B. halon
C. metal X
D. pressurized water

460. What are the contents of a multipurpose (ABC) fire extinguisher?

A. carbon dioxide
B. dry chemical
C. halon
D. metal X

461. If a specimen tube containing patient blood breaks in a centrifuge, what is the first thing the phlebotomist should do?

A. clean up the glass
B. spray the spill with disinfectant
C. sprinkle the spill with absorbent material
D. unplug the centrifuge

462. What are the three components of radiation safety?

A. alarm, confine, extinguish
B. PPE, engineering controls, education
C. stop, drop, roll
D. time, shielding, distance

463. Labeling of hazardous materials is required by:

A. OSHA's Bloodborne Pathogen Standard
B. OSHA's Hazardous Communication Standard
C. Patient's Bill of Rights
D. universal precautions

464. A form provided by chemical manufacturers containing general information, safe handling, and emergency information regarding a particular chemical is called a(n):

A. incident report
B. material safety data sheet
C. procedure manual
D. warning label

465. An agency that establishes standards for the operation of hospitals and other health care agencies, conducts surveys, and accredits programs that meet the defined standards is:

A. ASCP
B. JCAHO
C. OSHA
D. NAACLS

466. Appropriately maintaining a centrifuge is an example of what kind of safety?

A. chemical
B. electrical
C. mechanical
D. radioactive

467. Which of the following activities should NEVER occur in the laboratory?

A. calibration
B. eating
C. pipetting
D. quality control

468. A factor causing emotional or mental strain or tension is called:

A. basal state
B. diurnal rhythm
C. rest
D. stress

469. A patient suffering from disease or injury to the central nervous system would most likely be admitted to the:

A. geriatric unit
B. neurological unit
C. obstetrical unit
D. orthopedic unit

470. A patient suffering from a mental or an emotional disorder would most likely be admitted to the:

A. neurological unit
B. obstetric unit
C. pediatric unit
D. psychiatric unit

471. A patient experiencing complications related to pregnancy would most likely be admitted to the:

A. obstetrical unit
B. odontalgic unit
C. oncology unit
D. orthopedic unit

472. The field of medicine that specializes in the diagnosis and treatment of the elderly population is called:

A. geriatrics
B. oncology
C. proctology
D. rheumatology

473. The field of medicine that deals with the diagnosis and treatment of joint and tissue diseases is:

A. geriatrics
B. pediatrics
C. proctology
D. rheumatology

474. The medical specialty that deals with the diagnosis and treatment of disorders of the eye is:

A. obstetrics
B. ophthalmology
C. otolaryngology
D. orthopedics

475. The field of medicine that deals with the diagnosis and treatment of diseases of the ear, nose, and throat is:

A. obstetrics
B. ophthalmology
C. orthopedics
D. otolaryngology

476. The department of medicine that specializes in the diagnosis and treatment of disorders associated with male sexual and reproductive systems and renal system for both sexes is:

A. cardiology
B. dermatology
C. immunology
D. urology

477. The medical department that specializes in the diagnosis and treatment of disorders associated with the esophagus, stomach, and intestines is:

A. gastroenterology
B. proctology
C. nephrology
D. rheumatology

478. The medical department that specializes in the treatment of disorders associated with hormone production is:

A. endocrinology
B. gastroenterology
C. nephrology
D. urology

479. The department that uses radioactive materials to diagnose, treat, and monitor disease processes is:

A. medical imaging
B. nuclear medicine
C. occupational therapy
D. radiation therapy

480. The department that assists patients in becoming as independently active as possible, given the limitations of their physical or mental problems is:

A. occupational therapy
B. physical therapy
C. psychiatric therapy
D. radiation therapy

481. The department that works with the patient to eliminate his or her disability or to restore mental or physical abilities lost as a result of illness or accident is:

A. occupational therapy
B. physical therapy
C. psychiatric therapy
D. radiation therapy

482. A physician who specializes in the diagnosis of disease from laboratory test results is a:

A. pathologist
B. proctologist
C. rheumatologist
D. urologist

483. A laboratory professional who enters the field after obtaining a bachelor's degree, including a year or more of study in medical technology, is a:

A. certified laboratory assistant
B. pathologist
C. medical laboratory technician
D. medical technologist

484. A laboratory professional who enters the field after obtaining an associate's degree is a:

A. certified laboratory assistant
B. pathologist
C. medical laboratory technician
D. medical technologist

485. A laboratory professional trained in all aspects of blood specimen collection and transport is a:

A. pathologist
B. phlebotomist
C. medical laboratory technician
D. medical technologist

486. A laboratory professional who is responsible for the administration of a particular section of the laboratory is a(n):

A. administrative technologist
B. medical technologist
C. pathologist
D. technical supervisor

487. A technologist with an advanced degree and several years experience who is responsible for overseeing all operations involving physician and patient services is a(n):

A. administrative technologist
B. medical technologist
C. pathologist
D. technical supervisor

488. What is the highest administrative position on a standard organizational chart for the clinical laboratory?

A. administrative technologist
B. medical laboratory technician
C. medical technologist
D. technical supervisor

489. The rupturing or destruction of red blood cells, resulting in the release of hemoglobin into the fluid portion of the blood, is called:

A. hemoconcentration
B. hemolysis
C. hemostasis
D. homeostasis

490. The disease state resulting from the invasion of the body by a pathogenic microorganism is called:

A. infection
B. inflammation
C. inoculation
D. intrinsic

491. An infection acquired in a health care facility is called:

A. nosocomial
B. nosophobia
C. nosotoxicosis
D. nosotropic

492. An infection control program that includes monitoring specific patient population groups and classifications of infection is called:

A. surveillance
B. susceptibility
C. viability
D. virulence

493. The three components of the chain of infection are:

A. source, mode of transmission, susceptible host
B. source, mode of transmission, virulence
C. source, viability, virulence
D. source, viability, mode of transmission

494. An infection that can be transmitted from one person to another is called:

A. communicable
B. communicans
C. viable
D. virulent

495. The term used to communicate an organism's capability of living is:

A. viability
B. virulence
C. vicarious
D. villosity

496. The ability to overcome the defense mechanisms of the host is an organism's:

A. viability
B. vicarious
C. villosity
D. virulence

497. *Salmonella* organisms are examples of what component of the chain of infection?

A. means of transmission
B. nosocomial infection
C. source
D. susceptible host

498. Which of the following is an example of a mode of transmission in the chain of infection?

A. *Salmonella*
B. *Shigella*
C. patient suffering from AIDS
D. venipuncture needle

499. Which of the following is an example of a susceptible host in the chain of infection?

A. airborne droplets
B. patient afflicted with AIDS
C. *Salmonella*
D. venipuncture needle

500. Human hands are examples of which component of the chain of infection?

A. mode of transmission
B. nosocomial infection
C. source
D. susceptible host

501. Airborne droplets are examples of which component of the chain of infection?

A. mode of transmission
B. nosocomial infection
C. source
D. susceptible host

502. A patient undergoing immunosuppressive therapy prior to transplant is an example of which component of the chain of infection?

A. mode of transmission
B. nosocomial infection
C. source
D. susceptible host

503. Which of the following agencies first recommended universal precautions?

A. CAP
B. CDC
C. NAACLS
D. OSHA

504. Universal precautions prevent the spread of which of the following pathogens?

A. acid fast bacillus
B. blood-borne
C. respiratory
D. tuberculosis

505. The term "blood-borne pathogens" most commonly refers to:

A. HAV and HBV
B. HBV and HIV
C. HBV and *Treponema pallidum*
D. HBV and *Plasmodium falciparum*

506. Under universal precautions, which patients are considered potentially infectious?

A. all of them
B. none of them
C. patients infected with HBV
D. patients infected with HIV

507. A synonym for the term "barrier protection," as it applies to blood-borne pathogens, is:

A. body substance isolation
B. category-specific isolation
C. isolation procedures
D. personal protective equipment

508. Which of the following PPE is required if splashing of blood and body fluids is likely?

A. handwashing
B. masks
C. needle recapping
D. respirators

509. Which of the following practices is prohibited under universal precautions?

A. handwashing using an alcohol rinse solution
B. handwashing using a foam solution
C. recapping needles
D. wearing masks

510. Under universal precautions, when should a phlebotomist change gloves?

A. after every patient
B. after every second patient
C. after every third patient
D. only when soiled

511. Under universal precautions, when should a phlebotomist wash his or her hands?

A. after every patient, once gloves are removed
B. between patients, without removing gloves
C. only if the gloves are soiled
D. whenever the phlebotomist wants to

512. Which of the following agencies mandated universal precautions, superseding all other regulatory requirements?

A. CDC
B. CAP
C. NAACLS
D. OSHA

513. The physical transfer of a pathogenic microbe through close contact such as kissing is:

A. direct contact transmission
B. indirect contact transmission
C. vector transmission
D. vehicle transmission

514. Transfer of a pathogenic microbe via an inanimate object such as bed linen is:

A. direct contact transmission
B. indirect contact transmission
C. vector transmission
D. vehicle transmission

515. The transfer of a pathogenic organism through sneezing or coughing is called:

A. airborne transmission
B. indirect contact transmission
C. droplet contact transmission
D. vector transmission

516. Transfer of a pathogenic microbe via contaminated food or drugs is:

A. direct contact transmission
B. indirect contact transmission
C. vector transmission
D. vehicle transmission

517. Transfer of a pathogenic organism via an insect or animal is;

A. direct contact transmission
B. indirect contact transmission
C. vector transmission
D. vehicle transmission

518. The practice of separating patients with communicable infections from other patients and limiting their contact with health care workers and visitors is called:

A. ischemia
B. isolation
C. nosocomial
D. virulence

519. Which of the following isolation systems, established by the CDC, is based on a diagnosis of a communicable disease, and includes a category titled "AFB Isolation"?

A. category specific isolation
B. disease specific isolation
C. protective isolation
D. universal precautions

520. Which of the following isolation systems does not require a diagnosis of communicable disease?

A. category specific isolation
B. disease specific isolation
C. protective isolation
D. reverse isolation

521. A patient has an infection that is highly contagious and can be transmitted by direct contact and via airborne transmission. What isolation category would the patient be placed in?

A. contact
B. enteric
C. respiratory
D. strict

522. Before a phlebotomist enters the room of a patient in strict isolation, the phlebotomist should wear:

A. gloves, gown, and eyewear
B. gloves, gown, and mask
C. gown, mask, and eyewear
D. mask and gloves only

523. A patient is admitted to the hospital with chickenpox. What category of isolation would the patient be placed in?

A. contact
B. enteric
C. none
D. strict

524. A patient is admitted to a hospital with influenza. What category of isolation would the patient be placed in?

A. contact
B. enteric
C. none
D. strict

525. If a patient is in strict isolation, what color is the sign on the patient's door?

A. blue
B. brown
C. green
D. yellow

526. If a patient is in respiratory isolation, what color is the sign on the patient's door?

A. blue
B. brown
C. green
D. yellow

527. If a patient is diagnosed with *Haemophilus influenzae,* what isolation category would he or she be placed in?

A. contact isolation
B. drainage/secretion
C. respiratory
D. strict

528. A patient is diagnosed with an infection that may be spread by droplet contact or through the air. Which isolation category would the patient be placed in?

A. contact
B. drainage/secretion
C. enteric
D. respiratory

529. A patient is placed in enteric isolation. What color is the sign on the patient's door?

A. blue
B. brown
C. green
D. yellow

530. A phlebotomist approaches a patient's isolation room. To determine the appropriate protective clothing to wear into the patient's room, the phlebotomist should:

A. ask the patient's doctor
B. ask the patient's nurse
C. consult the sign on the patient's door
D. consult the Laboratory Procedure Manual

531. If a patient has an intestinal infection that can be spread by ingestion of the pathogen, which isolation category would the patient be placed in?

A. contact
B. enteric
C. respiratory
D. strict

532. If a patient is diagnosed with *Salmonella* infection, what isolation category would the patient be placed in?

A. contact
B. enteric
C. respiratory
D. strict

533. If a patient is placed in AFB isolation, what color is the sign on the patient's door?

A. brown
B. gray
C. orange
D. yellow

534. Which of the following personal protective equipment must a phlebotomist wear into a patient's room in AFB isolation?

A. gown and gloves
B. gloves and mask
C. gown, gloves, and mask
D. gown, gloves, and particulate respirator

535. If a patient is in AFB isolation, what diagnosis has been made?

A. *Haemophilus influenzae*
B. salmonellosis
C. shigellosis
D. tuberculosis

536. A patient is diagnosed with a highly transmissible disease that does not warrant strict isolation. What isolation category would the patient be placed in?

A. contact
B. drainage/secretion
C. enteric
D. respiratory

537. If a patient is diagnosed with a condition requiring drainage and secretion isolation, what color would the sign on the patient's door be?

A. blue
B. brown
C. green
D. yellow

538. A patient, burned over 75% of his body, develops an infection. What isolation category would he or she be placed in?

A. blood and body fluids
B. drainage/secretion
C. enteric
D. strict

539. Which category of isolation was replaced by universal precautions?

A. AFB isolation
B. blood and body fluids
C. contact isolation
D. enteric precautions

540. If a patient is undergoing immunosuppressive therapy prior to transplant, what isolation category would he be placed in?

A. contact
B. enteric
C. protective
D. strict

541. What procedure should be followed to dispose of trash and linens from an isolation room?

A. disinfection
B. double bagging
C. handwashing
D. reverse isolation

542. Chemical compounds used to remove or kill microorganisms on work surfaces or instruments are called:

A. aerosols
B. antiseptics
C. disinfectants
D. phloxine B

543. Chemicals that may be used on human skin to inhibit the growth and development of microorganisms, but not necessarily kill them, are:

A. aerosols
B. antiseptics
C. disinfectants
D. phenols

544. Which of the following is an antiseptic?

A. chloramine
B. formaldehyde
C. hypochlorite solution
D. 70% isopropyl alcohol

545. Which of the following compounds is a disinfectant?

A. 70% isopropyl alcohol
B. 1% phenol
C. hexachlorophene
D. quaternary ammonium compounds

546. Laboratory-acquired infections are often transmitted via:

A. respirator contact
B. skin contact
C. vector transmission
D. vehicle transmission

547. To prevent the spread of laboratory-acquired infections by ingestion, phlebotomists on duty should never:

A. handle a stick of gum
B. open centrifuges before they have stopped spinning
C. pop off the stoppers of evacuated tubes
D. rub their eyes

548. The phlebotomist enters a patient's room and realizes that the patient is not there. The phlebotomist should:

A. notify the doctor
B. notify the nurse
C. wait in the room for the patient to return
D. write "Can't get" on the requisition

549. If a patient refuses to have his blood drawn, the phlebotomist should *first:*

A. ask the nurse to try and enlist the patient's cooperation
B. politely leave the room
C. remind the patient that his or her physician ordered the test
D. write "Can't get" on the requisition

550. A patient refuses to have his blood drawn. The phlebotomist reminds the patient that his physician ordered the test, the patient still refuses; the phlebotomist should *next:*

A. ask the nurse to try and enlist the patient's cooperation
B. politely leave the room
C. remind the patient that his or her physician ordered the test
D. write "Can't get" on the requisition

551. The document adopted by the American Hospital Association in 1973 that protects the patient's right to refuse treatment is:

A. OSHA's Bloodborne Pathogen Standard
B. the Patient's Bill of Rights
C. the Right to Know Act
D. universal precautions

552. If a phlebotomist forcibly collects a blood specimen from a patient after the patient has refused the test, the phlebotomist can be charged with:

A. battery
B. malpractice
C. negligence
D. slander

553. The safety rules recommended by the CDC to prevent the spread of bloodborne pathogens are called:

A. epidemiology
B. isolation
C. protective isolation
D. universal precautions

554. Which of the following documents legally mandates precautions to minimize occupational exposure to bloodborne pathogens?

A. OSHA's Bloodborne Pathogen Standard
B. Patient's Bill of Rights
C. Phlebotomist Code of Ethics
D. universal precautions

555. Acquired immune deficiency syndrome is associated with:

A. HAV
B. HBV
C. HCV
D. HIV

556. The use of body language in communication is called:

A. kinesics
B. proxemics
C. sign language
D. unprofessional

557. A method of nonverbal communication involving a person's use and concept of space is called:

A. body language
B. kinesics
C. proxemics
D. unprofessional

558. Requisitions for laboratory testing originate with the patient's

A. nurse
B. patient care associate
C. physician
D. respiratory therapist

559. Which of the following instruments is most frequently used for two-way communication?

A. computer
B. memoranda
C. procedure manual
D. telephone

560. Which of the following systems is most error-free in making requests to the laboratory for test procedures?

A. computer-generated requisitions
B. key punch generated requisitions
C. manually written requisitions
D. verbal requisitions

561. The term applied to communication barriers, as diagramed in the communication loop, is:

A. feedback
B. filter
C. receiver
D. sender

562. When verbal and nonverbal messages do not match, it is called:

A. empathy
B. filter
C. kinesic slip
D. proxemic slip

563. An example of positive body language is:

A. chewing gum
B. smiling
C. staring
D. tapping foot

564. An example of negative body language is:

A. chewing gum
B. erect posture
C. maintaining eye contact
D. smiling

565. The term that applies to a program that guarantees quality patient care is:

A. quality assurance
B. quality control
C. continuous quality improvement
D. total quality management

566. The term used to denote specific procedures within a program designed to ensure quality patient care is:

A. quality assurance
B. quality control
C. continuous quality improvement
D. total quality management

567. A system of evaluation mandated by JCAHO that targets healthcare outcomes and processes for improvement is called:

A. quality assurance
B. quality control
C. continuous quality improvement
D. total quality management

568. According to NCCLS, draw volumes of evacuated tubes must be within what range of the scheduled draw?

A. +/– 3%
B. +/– 5%
C. +/– 7%
D. +/– 10%

569. A phlebotomist is scheduled to collect 7 mL of specimen in an evacuated tube. According to NCCLS, what is the acceptable range of draw volume?

A. 6.8 to 7.2 mL
B. 6.7 to 7.4 mL
C. 6.5 to 7.5 mL
D. 6.3 to 7.7 mL

570. A phlebotomist selects a needle for a venipuncture procedure. She notices that the seal surrounding the needle is loosened. The phlebotomist should:

A. discard the needle
B. notify security
C. notify her supervisor
D. use the needle

571. A device used to measure RPMs (rotations per minute) on centrifuges is called a(n):

A. aneroid gauge
B. refractometer
C. sphygmomanometer
D. tachometer

572. When testing blood pressure cuffs for slow leaks, the mercury should not change by more than what rate to be acceptable?

A. 1 mm Hg/sec
B. 3 mm Hg/sec
C. 5 mm Hg/sec
D. 7 mm Hg/sec

573. To ensure quality bleeding time results by the modified Ivy bleeding time method, the blood pressure cuff should be inflated to what reading?

A. 10 mm Hg
B. 20 mm Hg
C. 30 mm Hg
D. 40 mm Hg

574. In addition to technical duties, the phlebotomist also is responsible for being the laboratory's:

A. QA officer
B. QC officer
C. public health representative
D. public relations representative

575. A patient will often equate his encounter with the phlebotomist with the:

A. caliber of care he is receiving
B. quality of the food
C. safety of his surroundings
D. skill of his physician

576. An adult quadriplegic patient refuses to have his blood drawn. The phlebotomist ignores his remark, and takes his blood, per the doctor's order. The phlebotomist can be charged with:

A. assault and battery
B. criminal abuse
C. nothing
D. malpractice

577. Civil lawsuit based on improper treatment or negligence by a professional person is called:

A. assault and battery
B. malpractice
C. negligence
D. respondeat superior

578. Failure to exercise reasonable skill in performing a task is called:

A. assault and battery
B. malpractice
C. negligence
D. respondeat superior

579. The concept that is commonly referred to as "Let the master answer," whereby a laboratory corporation can be held responsible for a laboratory worker's negligent action, is:

A. assault and battery
B. malpractice
C. negligence
D. respondeat superior

580. A person who is legally responsible for damages assigned in a legal action is called:

A. defendant
B. liable
C. felon
D. tort

581. The term referring to a civil wrong, in which the person committing the wrong is responsible for damages, is called:

A. liability
B. malpractice
C. negligence
D. tort

582. The case law that awards damages based on negligence of the laboratory in performing blood typing is:

A. Helmann v. Sacred Heart
B. Lazernick v. General Hospital of Monroe County
C. Paros v. Hoemako Hospital
D. Schmerber v. State of California

583. A claim that can be filed by a patient, due to unauthorized release of personal information, is called:

A. assault
B. invasion of privacy
C. malpractice
D. respondeat superior

584. Which of the following would be classified as an engineering control, according to OSHA's Bloodborne Pathogen Standard?

A. gloves
B. gown
C. handwashing
D. self-sheathing needle

585. Hemogard™ closures of evacuated tubes prevent:

A accidental self-puncture with a contaminated needle
B. aerosal formation upon stopper removal
D. hemoconcentration
D. hemolysis

586. Which of the following test procedures requires the same patient identification procedures as a type and crossmatch?

A. group and Rh
B. platelet count
C. *Toxoplasma* antibody screen
D. type and screen

587. Blood may be collected from a patient without a standard hospital identification bracelet if the patient is in which of the following circumstances?

A. emergency department
B. operating room
C. pediatric department
D. recovery room

588. Which of the following is ensured to the patient by the Patient's Bill of Rights?

A. adequate parking for visitors
B. adherence to proper patient identification procedures
C. medical records will remain confidential
D. prompt response to call lights

589. What is the most important step in any blood collection procedure to ensure quality results?

A. patient approach
B. patient identification
C. patient preparation
D. post-phlebotomy patient care

CHAPTER 5

Images

590. The above symbol warns of a:

   A. carcinogen hazard
   B. corrosive hazard
   C. flammable hazard
   D. radiation hazard

591. The above symbol warns of a:

   A. carcinogen hazard
   B. corrosive hazard
   C. flammable hazard
   D. radiation hazard

592. The symbol pictured above warns of a:

A. carcinogen hazard
B. corrosive hazard
C. flammable hazard
D. radiation hazard

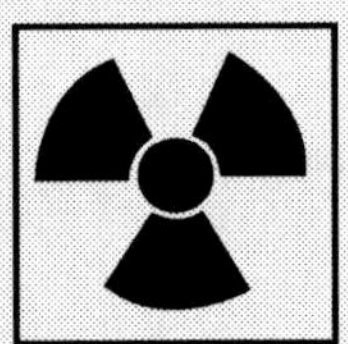

593. The symbol pictured above warns of a:

A. carcinogen hazard
B. corrosive hazard
C. flammable hazard
D. radiation hazard

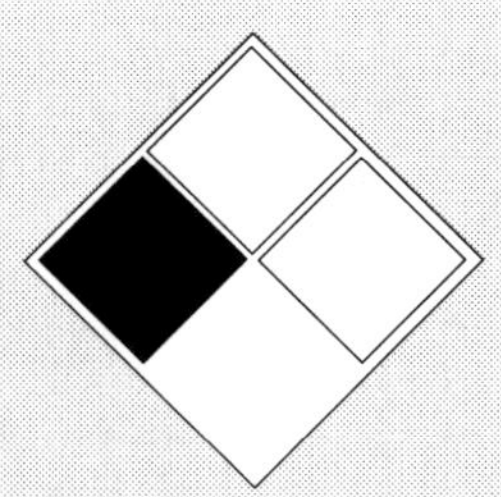

594. The above symbol is the:

A. DOT hazardous material label
B. NFPA chemical hazard sign
C. material safety data sheet
D. Nuclear Regulatory Commission symbol

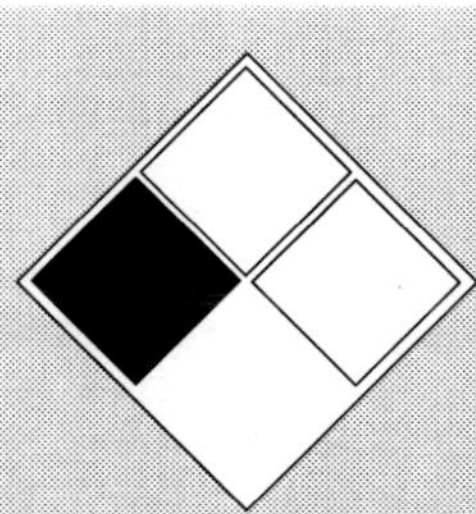

595. On the symbol above, what color is the diamond on the top?

A. blue
B. red
C. yellow
D. white

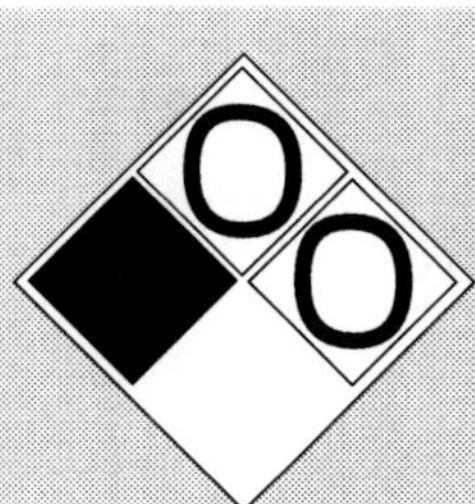

596. On the symbol above, the diamond on the right warns of a:

A. flammability hazard
B. health hazard
C. instability hazard
D. radioactive hazard

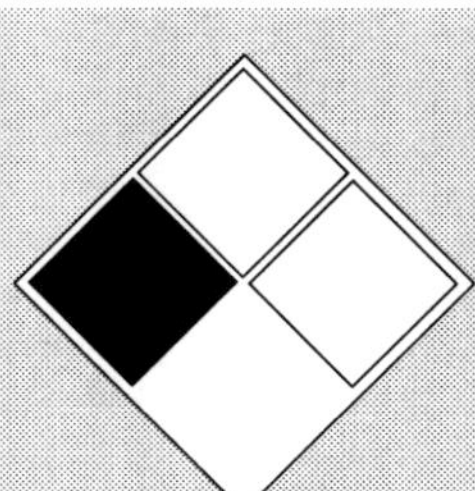

597. On the symbol above, the diamond on the left warns of a:

A. flammability hazard
B. health hazard
C. instability hazard
D. radioactive hazard

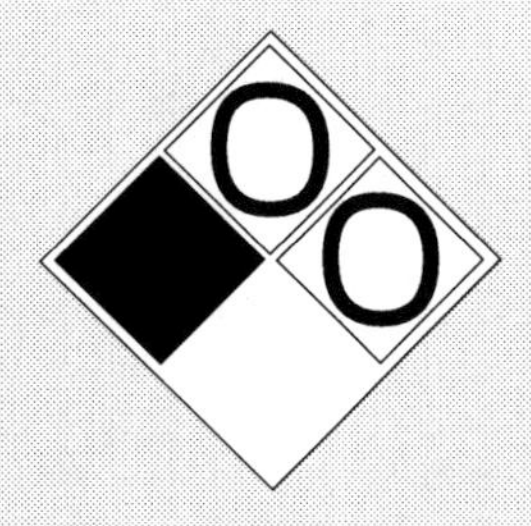

598. In the symbol above, the number "0" in the diamond on the right communicates:

A. explosive at room temperature
B. extremely flammable
C. no health hazard
D. not reactive when mixed with water

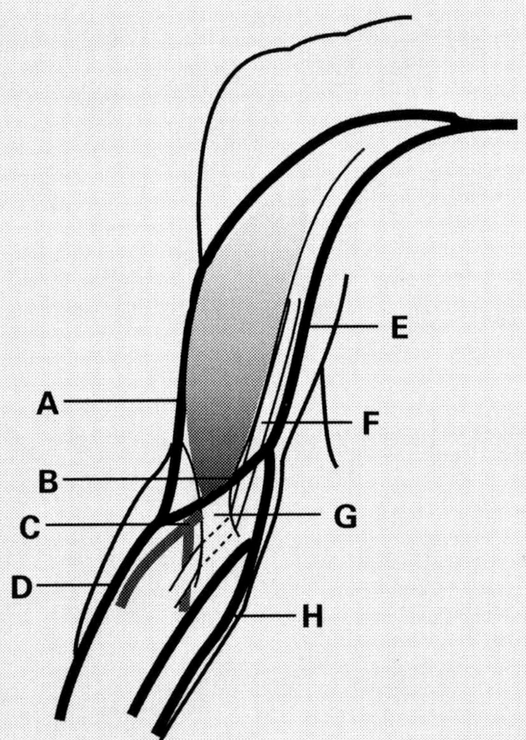

599. Please refer to the above diagram to answer the next eight questions. Identify structure A in the diagram.

A. basilic vein
B. brachial artery
C. cephalic vein
D. median cubital vein

600. Identify structure B in the diagram.

A. basilic vein
B. brachial artery
C. cephalic vein
D. median cubital vein

601. Identify structure C in the diagram.

A. basilic vein
B. brachial artery
C. cephalic vein
D. median cubital vein

602. Identify structure D in the diagram.

A. basilic vein
B. brachial artery
C. cephalic vein
D. median cubital vein

603. Identify structure E in the diagram.

A. basilic vein
B. bicipital aponeurosis
C. cephalic vein
D. median nerve

604. Identify structure F in the diagram.

A. basilic vein
B. bicipital aponeurosis
C. cephalic vein
D. median nerve

605. Identify structure G in the diagram.

A. basilic vein
B. bicipital aponeurosis
C. cephalic vein
D. median nerve

606. Identify structure H in the diagram.

A. basilic vein
B. bicipital aponeurosis
C. cephalic vein
D. median nerve

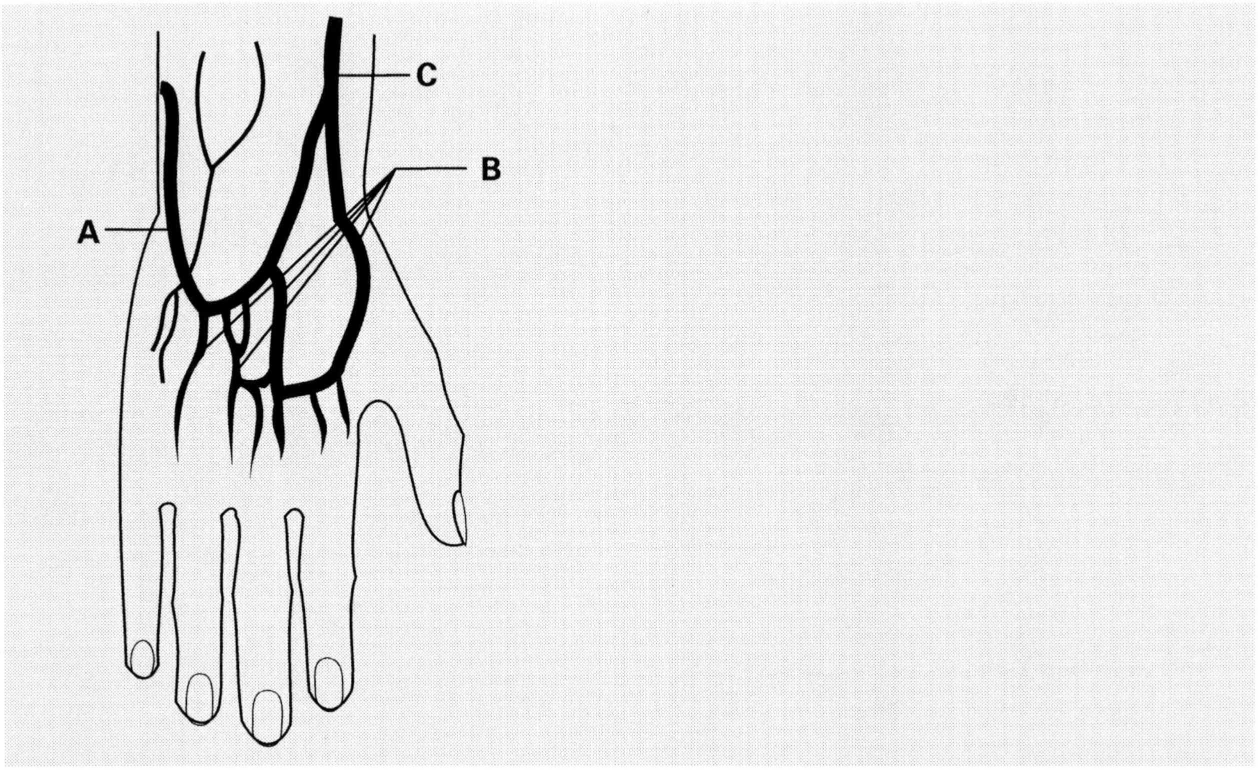

607. Please refer to the above diagram to answer the next three questions. Identify structure A in the diagram.

A. basilic vein
B. cephalic vein
C. dorsal metacarpal veins
D. median cubital vein

608. Identify structure B in the diagram.

A. basilic vein
B. cephalic vein
C. dorsal metacarpal vein
D. median cubital vein

609. Identify structure C in the diagram.

A. basilic vein
B. cephalic vein
C. dorsal metacarpal veins
D. median cubital vein

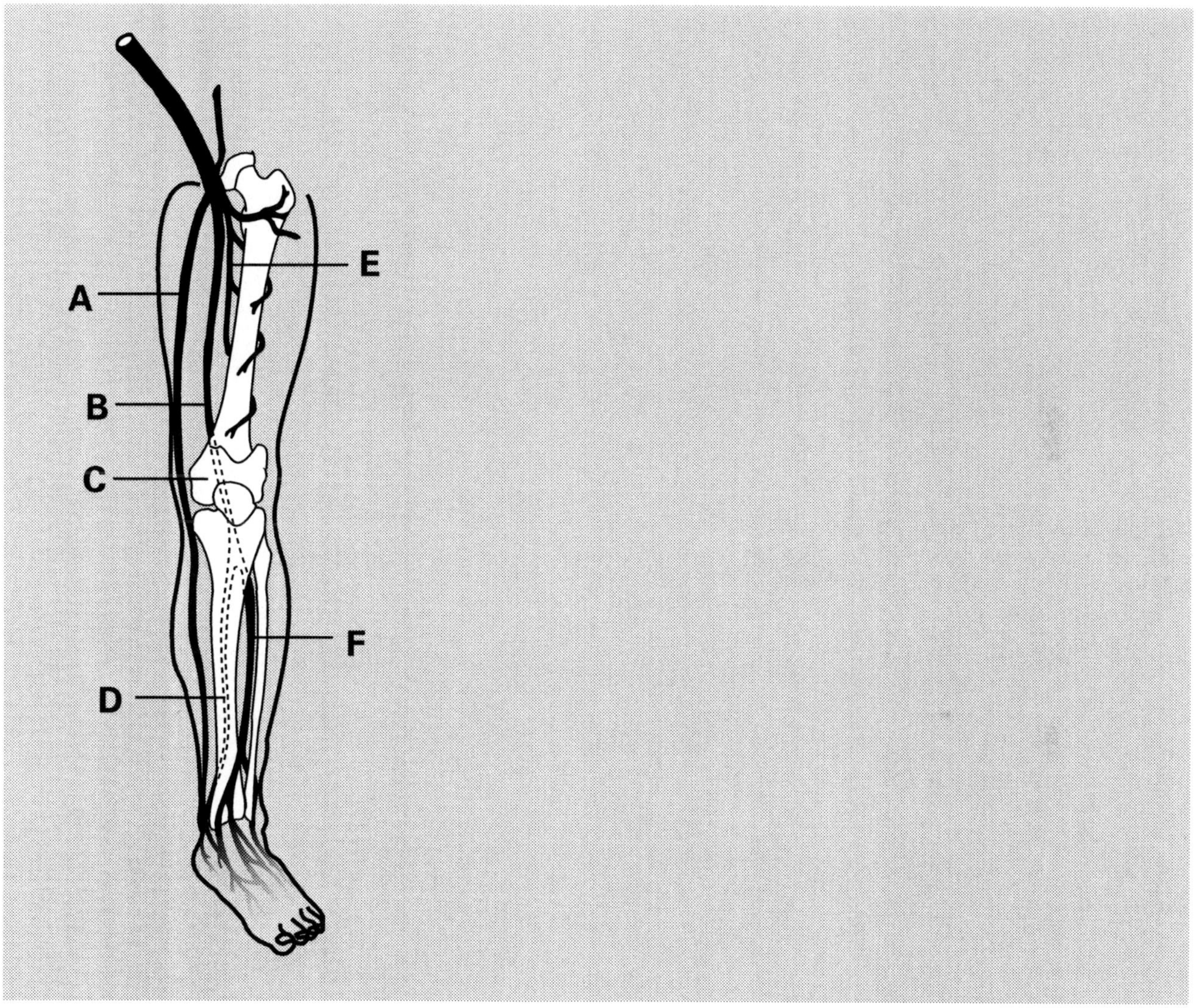

610. Please refer to the above diagram to answer the next two questions. Identify structure A in the diagram.

A. deep femoral vein
B. femoral vein
C. great saphenous vein
D. popliteal vein

611. Identify structure B in the diagram.

A. deep femoral vein
B. femoral vein
C. great saphenous vein
D. popliteal vein

612. Identify the piece of equipment pictured above.

A. autolet
B. hemalet
C. Safety flow lancet™
D. Tenderfoot™

613. Identify the piece of equipment pictured above.

A. autolet
B. hemalet
C. Safety flow lancet™
D. Tenderfoot™

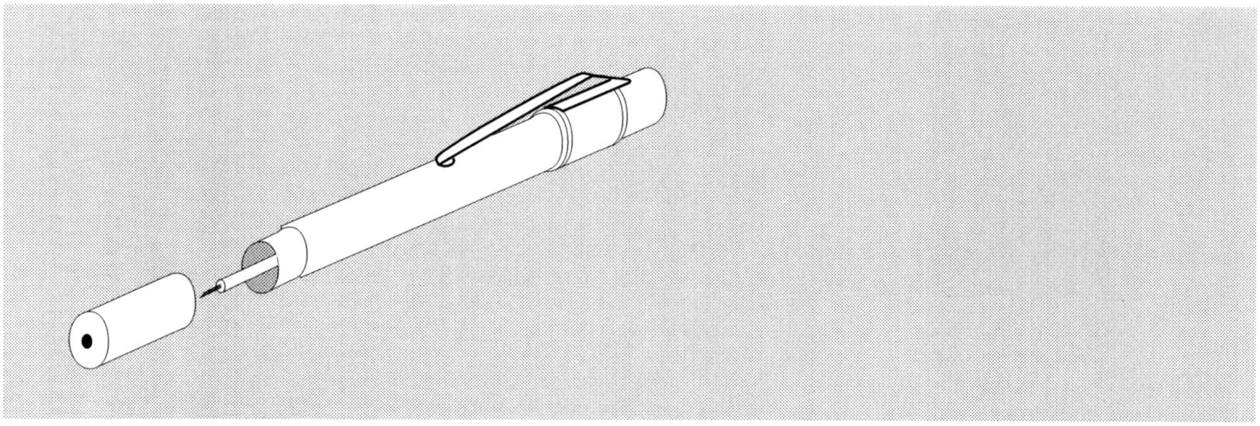

614. Identify the piece of equipment pictured above.

A. autolet
B. hemalet
C. Safety flow lancet™
D. Tenderfoot™

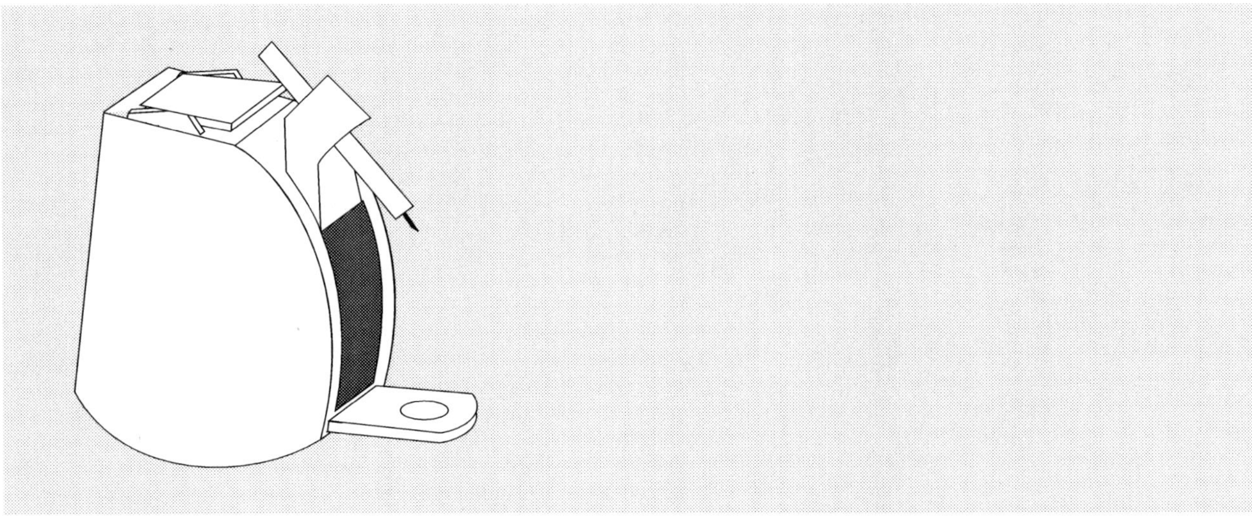

615. Identify the piece of equipment pictured above.

A. autolet
B. hemalet
C. Safety flow lancet™
D. Tenderfoot™

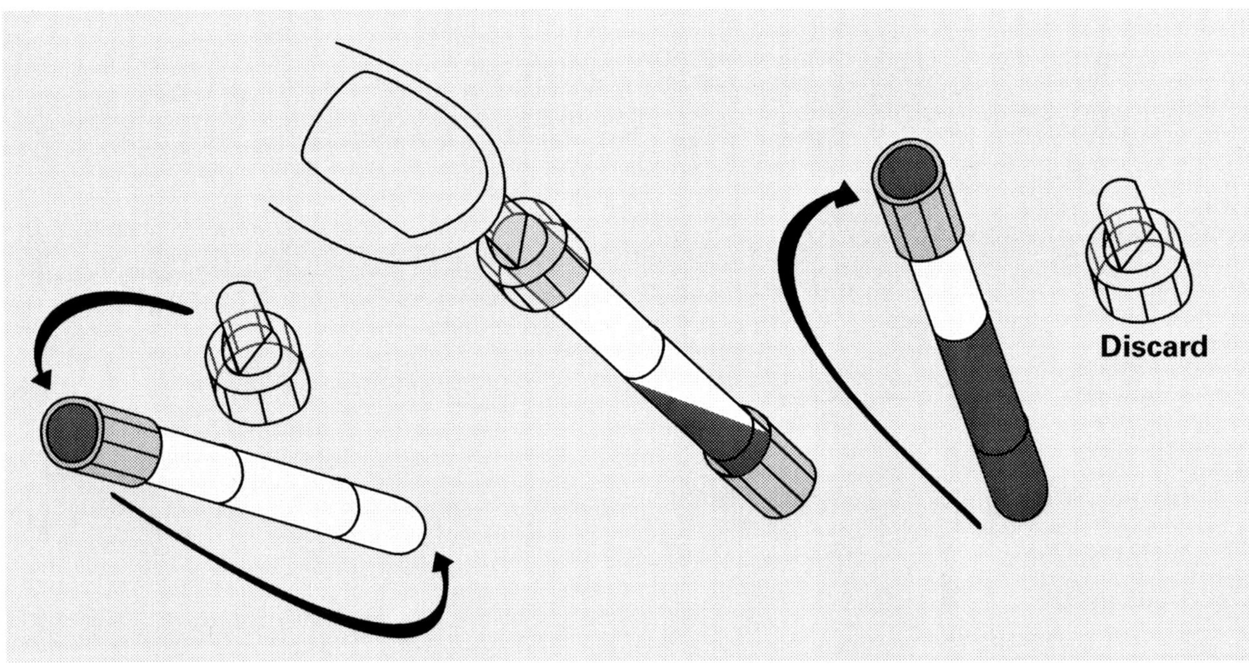

616. Identify the piece of equipment pictured above.

A. evacuated tube system
B. microhematocrit capillary tubes
C. Microtainer™ collector
D. Unopette™ system

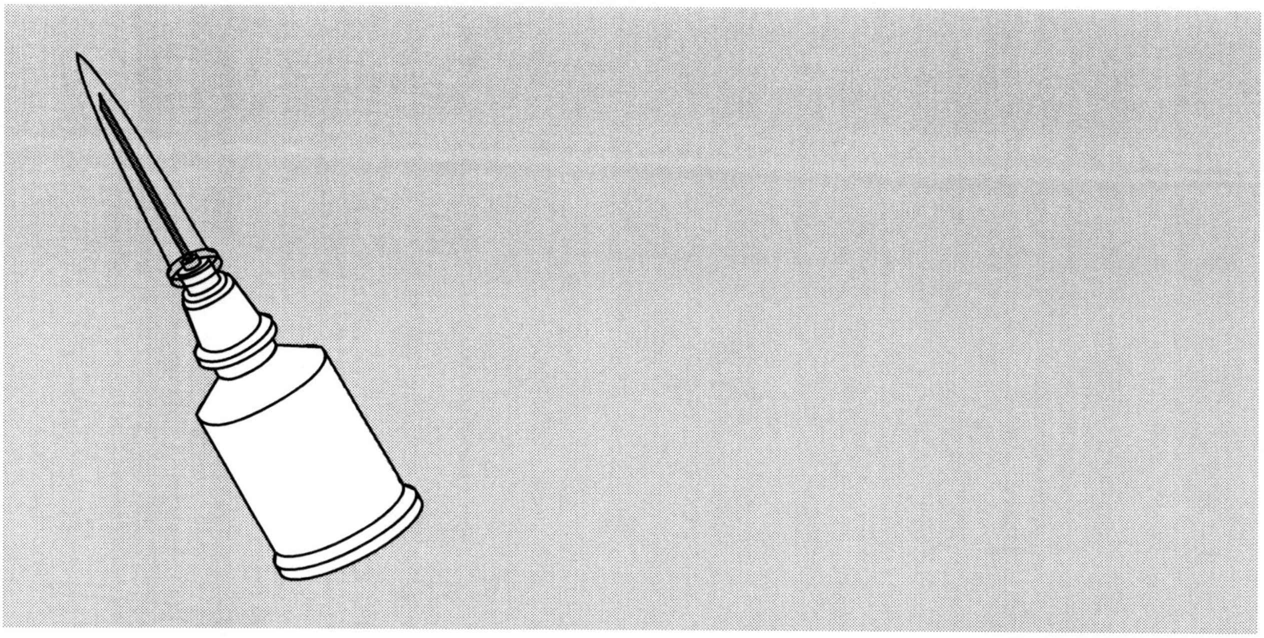

617. Identify the piece of equipment pictured above.

A. evacuated tube system
B. microhematocrit capillary tubes
C. Microtainer™ collector
D. Unopette™ system

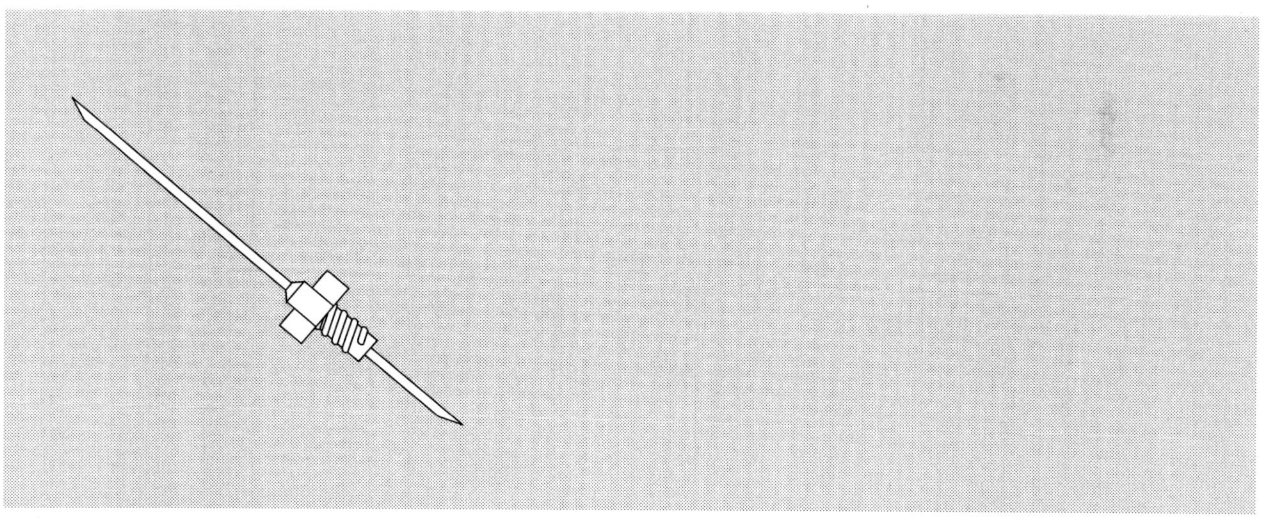

618. Identify the piece of equipment pictured above.

A. Microtainer™
B. multisample needle
C. single sample needle
D. syringe needle

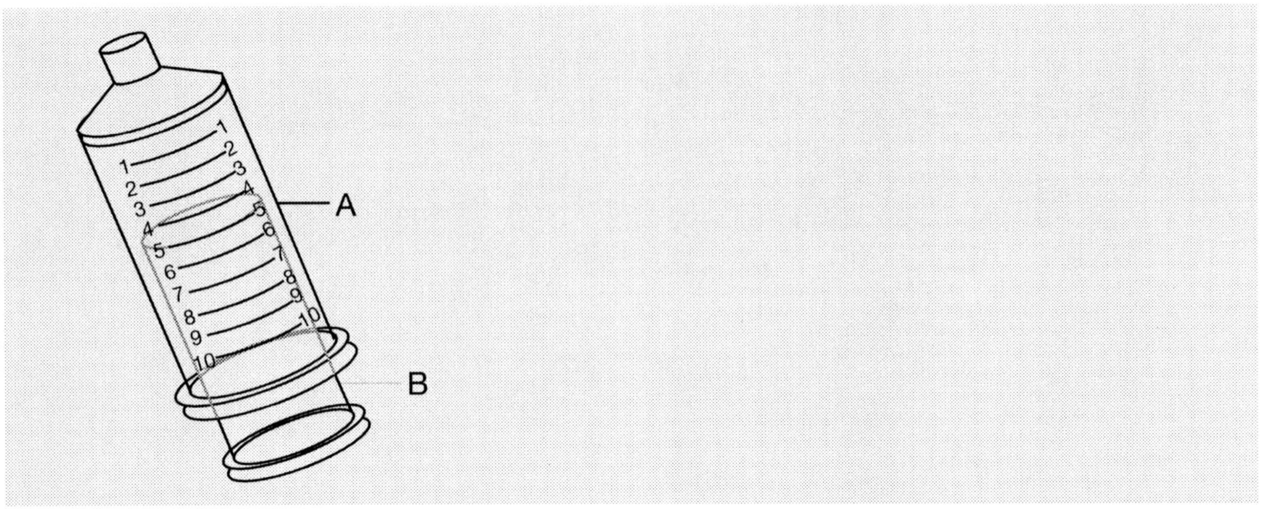

619. Pictured above is a piece of equipment. Identify the part labeled "A."

A. barrel
B. bevel
C. plunger
D. shaft

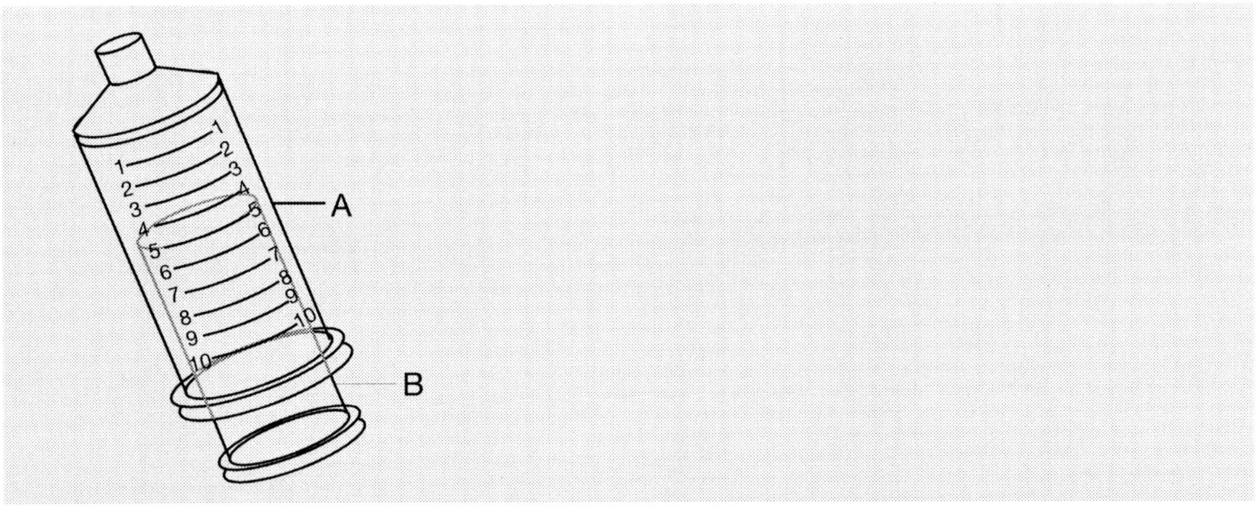

620. Pictured above is a piece of equipment. Identify the part labeled "B."

A. barrel
B. bevel
C. plunger
D. shaft

621. Pictured above is a piece of equipment. Identify the part labeled "A."

A. barrel
B. bevel
C. hub
D. shaft

622. Pictured above is a piece of equipment. Identify the part labeled "C."

A. barrel
B. bevel
C. hub
D. shaft

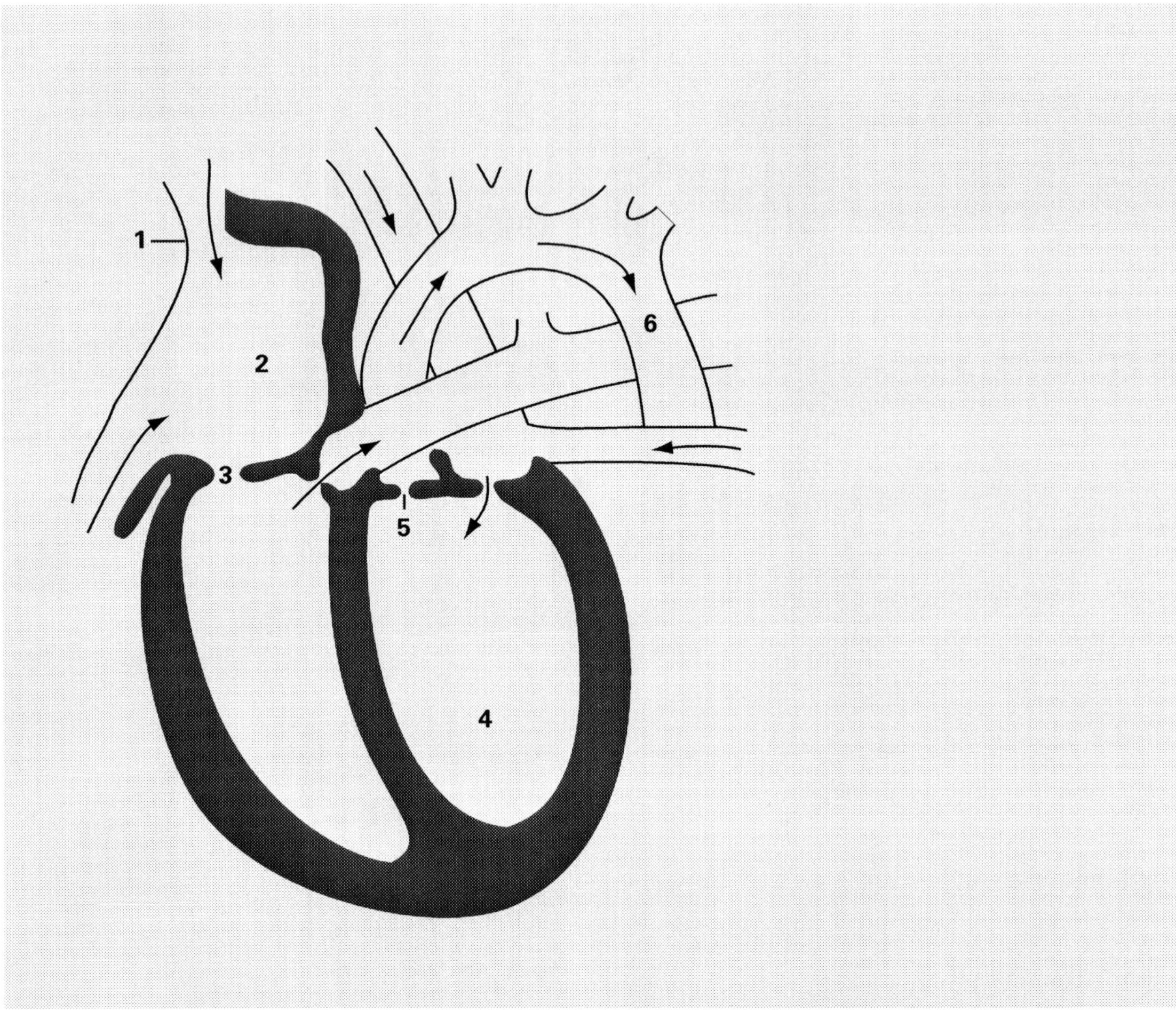

623. Please use the above diagram to answer the next six questions. Identify the structure labeled "1" on the diagram.

A. aorta
B. inferior vena cava
C. superior vena cava
D. pulmonary vein

624. Identify the structure labeled "6" on the diagram.

A. aorta
B. inferior vena cava
C. superior vena cava
D. pulmonary vein

625. Identify the structure labeled "4" on the diagram.

A. right atrium
B. left atrium
C. right ventricle
D. left ventricle

626. Identify the structure labeled "2" on the diagram.

A. right atrium
B. left atrium
C. right ventricle
D. left ventricle

627. Identify the structure labeled "3" on the diagram.

A. bicuspid valve
B. tricuspid valve
C. aortic valve
D. pulmonic valve

628. Identify the structure labeled "5" on the diagram.

A. bicuspid valve
B. tricuspid valve
C. aortic valve
D. pulmonic valve

Answer Key

1. **D**
   Phlebotomy Essentials, p. 62
2. **D**
   Phlebotomy Handbook, Fourth Ed., p. 43
3. **D**
   Phlebotomy Essentials, p. 61
4. **B**
   Phlebotomy Handbook, Fourth Ed., p. 43
5. **A**
   Phlebotomy Handbook, Fourth Ed., p. 43
6. **C**
   Phlebotomy Essentials, p. 58
7. **A**
   Phlebotomy Essentials, p. 58
8. **D**
   Phlebotomy Essentials, p. 58
9. **A**
   Phlebotomy Essentials, p. 59
10. **D**
    Phlebotomy Essentials, p. 59
11. **D**
    Phlebotomy Essentials, p. 59
12. **A**
    Phlebotomy Essentials, p. 59
13. **C**
    Phlebotomy Essentials, p. 59
14. **B**
    Phlebotomy Essentials, p. 59
15. **D**
    Phlebotomy Essentials, p. 60
16. **A**
    Phlebotomy Essentials, p. 60
17. **C**
    Phlebotomy Essentials, p. 60
18. **B**
    Phlebotomy Essentials, p. 60
19. **B**
    Phlebotomy Essentials, p. 60
20. **A**
    Phlebotomy Essentials, p. 60
21. **D**
    Phlebotomy Essentials, p. 58
22. **A**
    Phlebotomy Essentials, p. 58
23. **B**
    Phlebotomy Essentials, p. 60
24. **A**
    Phlebotomy Essentials, p. 60
25. **B**
    Phlebotomy Essentials, p. 60
26. **D**
    Phlebotomy Essentials, p. 60
27. **A**
    Phlebotomy Essentials, p. 60
28. **C**
    Phlebotomy Essentials, p. 60
29. **A**
    Phlebotomy Essentials, p. 93
30. **D**
    Phlebotomy Essentials, p. 58

31. **D**
Phlebotomy Essentials, p. 58

32. **D**
Phlebotomy Essentials, p. 58

33. **A**
Phlebotomy Essentials, p. 101

34. **D**
Phlebotomy Essentials, p. 103

35. **B**
Phlebotomy Essentials, p. 102

36. **B**
Phlebotomy Essentials, p. 102

37. **C**
Phlebotomy Essentials, p. 103

38. **C**
Phlebotomy Essentials, p. 105

39. **A**
Phlebotomy Essentials, p. 105

40. **C**
Phlebotomy Essentials, p. 107

41. **A**
Phlebotomy Essentials, p. 107

42. **B**
Phlebotomy Essentials, p. 108

43. **A**
Phlebotomy Essentials, p. 108

44. **A**
Phlebotomy Essentials, pp. 107 and 108

45. **D**
Phlebotomy Essentials, p. 109

46. **C**
Phlebotomy Essentials, p. 73

47. **B**
Phlebotomy Essentials, p. 64

48. **A**
Phlebotomy Essentials, p. 68

49. **B**
Phlebotomy Essentials, p. 66

50. **D**
Phlebotomy Essentials, p. 77

51. **C**
Phlebotomy Essentials, pp. 81 and 82

52. **A**
Phlebotomy Essentials, p. 70

53. **C**
Phlebotomy Essentials, p. 95

54. **D**
Phlebotomy Essentials, p. 95

55. **B**
Phlebotomy Essentials, p. 95

56. **A**
Phlebotomy Essentials, p. 93

57. **B**
Phlebotomy Essentials, p. 88

58. **A**
Phlebotomy Essentials, p. 96

59. **D**
Phlebotomy Essentials, p. 96

60. **A**
Phlebotomy Essentials, p. 93

61. **D**
Phlebotomy Handbook, Fourth Ed., p. 330

62. **B**
Phlebotomy Handbook, Fourth Ed., p. 330

63. **B**
Phlebotomy Handbook, Fourth Ed., p. 328

64. **B**
Urinalysis and Body Fluids, p. 172

65. **D**
Phlebotomy Essentials, p. 96

66. **A**
Phlebotomy Essentials, p. 97

67. **D**
Phlebotomy Essentials, p. 96

68. **C**
Phlebotomy Essentials, p. 97

69. **D**
Phlebotomy Essentials, Color Plate 1

70. **A**
Phlebotomy Essentials, Color Plate 1

71. **C**
Phlebotomy Handbook, Fourth Ed., p. 79

72. **A**
Phlebotomy Handbook, Fourth Ed., p. 80

73. **B**
Handbook of Phlebotomy, Third Ed., p. 52

74. **A**
Phlebotomy Essentials, p. 298

75. **D**
Phlebotomy Techniques: A Laboratory Workbook, p. 202

76. **B**
Phlebotomy Handbook, Fourth Ed., p. 251

77. **A**
Phlebotomy Essentials, p. 157

78. **B**
Phlebotomy Essentials, p. 158

79. **C**
Phlebotomy Essentials, p. 157

80. **C**
Phlebotomy Techniques: A Laboratory Workbook, p. 34

81. **A**
Phlebotomy Essentials, Color Plate 2

82. **C**
Phlebotomy Essentials, Color Plate 2

83. **B**
Phlebotomy Essentials, Color Plate 2

84. **B**
Handbook of Phlebotomy, Third Ed., p. 54

85. **C**
Phlebotomy Essentials, Color Plate 2

86. **D**
Phlebotomy Essentials, Color Plate 2

87. **D**
Phlebotomy Essentials, Color Plate 2

88. **B**
Phlebotomy Essentials, Color Plate 2

89. **C**
Phlebotomy Techniques: A Laboratory Workbook, p. 35

90. **C**
Phlebotomy Techniques: A Laboratory Workbook, p. 35

91. **C**
Phlebotomy Essentials, Color Plate 2

92. **A**
Phlebotomy Essentials, Color Plate 2

93. **C**
Phlebotomy Essentials, Color Plate 2

94. **A**
Phlebotomy Techniques: A Laboratory Workbook, p. 268

95. **D**
Phlebotomy Essentials, Color Plate 2

96. **A**
Phlebotomy Techniques: A Laboratory Workbook, p. 35

97. **D**
Phlebotomy Essentials, Color Plate 2

98. **C**
Phlebotomy Essentials, p. 157

99. **D**
Phlebotomy Essentials, p. 157

100. **A**
Phlebotomy Essentials, p. 157

101. **D**
Phlebotomy Essentials, p. 157

102. **C**
Phlebotomy Techniques: A Laboratory Workbook, p. 35

103. **B**
Phlebotomy Techniques: A Laboratory Workbook, p. 35

104. **B**
Phlebotomy Handbook, Fourth Ed., p. 126

105. **D**
Phlebotomy Essentials, Color Plate 2

106. **A**
Phlebotomy Techniques: A Laboratory Workbook, p. 35

107. **C**
Phlebotomy Techniques: A Laboratory Workbook, p. 35

108. **C**
Phlebotomy Techniques: A Laboratory Workbook, p. 35

109. **D**
Handbook of Phlebotomy, Third Ed., p. 65

110. **B**
Handbook of Phlebotomy, Third Ed., p. 65

111. **D**
Handbook of Phlebotomy, Third Ed., p. 65

112. **D**
Phlebotomy Techniques: A Laboratory Workbook, p. 133

113. **C**
Phlebotomy Essentials, p. 239

114. **B**
Phlebotomy Essentials, p. 239

115. **C**
Phlebotomy Techniques: A Laboratory Workbook, p. 265

116. **C**
Phlebotomy Essentials, p. 251

117. **B**
Phlebotomy Essentials, p. 176

118. **A**
Phlebotomy Essentials, p. 176

119. **A**
Phlebotomy Essentials, p. 176

120. **B**
Phlebotomy Essentials, p. 176

121. **A**
Phlebotomy Essentials, p. 176

122. **D**
Phlebotomy Essentials, p. 176

123. **D**
Phlebotomy Essentials, p. 177

124. **C**
Phlebotomy Essentials, p. 178

125. **A**
Phlebotomy Essentials, p. 178

126. **D**
Phlebotomy Essentials, p. 178

127. **B**
Phlebotomy Essentials, p. 178

128. **C**
Phlebotomy Essentials, p. 239

129. **C**
Phlebotomy Essentials, p. 239

130. **D**
Phlebotomy Essentials, p. 239

131. **C**
Phlebotomy Essentials, p. 239

132. **C**
Phlebotomy Essentials, p. 239

133. **C**
Phlebotomy Essentials, p. 238

134. **A**
Phlebotomy Techniques: A Laboratory Workbook, p. 224

135. **B**
Phlebotomy Essentials, p. 239

136. **C**
Phlebotomy Essentials, p. 239

137. **A**
Phlebotomy Essentials, p. 239

138. **D**
Phlebotomy Handbook, Fourth Ed., p. 481

139. **B**
Phlebotomy Essentials, p. 5

140. **B**
Phlebotomy Essentials, p. 198

141. **C**
Phlebotomy Essentials, p. 198

142. **B**
Phlebotomy Essentials, p. 199

143. **A**
Phlebotomy Essentials, p. 199

144. **A**
Phlebotomy Essentials, p. 199

145. **B**
Phlebotomy Essentials, p. 199

146. **B**
Phlebotomy Techniques: A Laboratory Workbook, p. 44

147. **C**
Phlebotomy Techniques: A Laboratory Workbook, p. 44

148. **D**
Phlebotomy Techniques: A Laboratory Workbook, p. 44

149. **D**
Phlebotomy Essentials, p. 200

150. **C**
Phlebotomy Essentials, p. 201

151. **A**
Phlebotomy Essentials, p. 201

152. **D**
Phlebotomy Techniques: A Laboratory Workbook, pp. xvii and xviii

153. **A**
Phlebotomy Techniques: A Laboratory Workbook, p. 47

154. **D**
Phlebotomy Techniques: A Laboratory Workbook, p. 47

155. **A**
Phlebotomy Essentials, p. 240

156. **C**
Phlebotomy Techniques: A Laboratory Workbook, p. 45

157. **D**
Phlebotomy Techniques: A Laboratory Workbook, p. 45

158. **C**
Phlebotomy Techniques: A Laboratory Workbook, p. 46

159. **C**
Phlebotomy Techniques: A Laboratory Workbook, p. 46

160. **D**
Phlebotomy Techniques: A Laboratory Workbook, p. 46

161. **D**
Phlebotomy Techniques: A Laboratory Workbook, p. 46

162. **B**
Phlebotomy Essentials, p. 242

163. **D**
Phlebotomy Essentials, p. 242

164. **A**
Phlebotomy Essentials, p. 242

165. **A**
Phlebotomy Essentials, p. 242

166. **C**
Phlebotomy Essentials, p. 242

167. **D**
Phlebotomy Techniques: A Laboratory Workbook, p. 97

168. **D**
Phlebotomy Techniques: A Laboratory Workbook, p. 126

169. **C**
Phlebotomy Techniques: A Laboratory Workbook, p. 126

170. **A**
Phlebotomy Techniques: A Laboratory Workbook, p. 126

171. **B**
Phlebotomy Techniques: A Laboratory Workbook, p. 136

172. **B**
Phlebotomy Techniques: A Laboratory Workbook, p. 136

173. **A**
Phlebotomy Techniques: A Laboratory Workbook, p. 136

174. **C**
Phlebotomy Techniques: A Laboratory Workbook, p. 63

175. **D**
Phlebotomy Techniques: A Laboratory Workbook, p. 63

176. **A**
Phlebotomy Techniques: A Laboratory Workbook, p. 63

177. **B**
Phlebotomy Techniques: A Laboratory Workbook, p. 63

178. **B**
Phlebotomy Techniques: A Laboratory Workbook, p. 63

179. **D**
Phlebotomy Techniques: A Laboratory Workbook, p. 64

180. **C**
Phlebotomy Techniques: A Laboratory Workbook, p. 64

181. **A**
Phlebotomy Techniques: A Laboratory Workbook, p. 67

182. **A**
Phlebotomy Techniques: A Laboratory Workbook, p. 67

183. **A**
Phlebotomy Techniques: A Laboratory Workbook, p. 66

184. **B**
Phlebotomy Techniques: A Laboratory Workbook, p. 65

185. **D**
Phlebotomy Techniques: A Laboratory Workbook, p. 63

186. **B**
Phlebotomy Techniques: A Laboratory Workbook, p. 74

187. **C**
Phlebotomy Techniques: A Laboratory Workbook, p. 74

188. **C**
Phlebotomy Techniques: A Laboratory Workbook, p. 74

189. **C**
Phlebotomy Techniques: A Laboratory Workbook, p. 74

190. **B**
Phlebotomy Techniques: A Laboratory Workbook, p. 62

191. **D**
Phlebotomy Techniques: A Laboratory Workbook, p. 74

192. **A**
Phlebotomy Techniques: A Laboratory Workbook, p. 74

193. **A**
Phlebotomy Techniques: A Laboratory Workbook, p. 73

194. **C**
Phlebotomy Techniques: A Laboratory Workbook, p. 73

195. **C**
Phlebotomy Techniques: A Laboratory Workbook, p. 77

196. **C**
Phlebotomy Techniques: A Laboratory Workbook, p. 77

197. **A**
Phlebotomy Techniques: A Laboratory Workbook, p. 76

198. **B**
Phlebotomy Techniques: A Laboratory Workbook, p. 77

199. **B**
Phlebotomy Techniques: A Laboratory Workbook, p. 77

200. **B**
Phlebotomy Techniques: A Laboratory Workbook, p. 75

201. **C**
Phlebotomy Techniques: A Laboratory Workbook, p. 77

202. **B**
Phlebotomy Essentials, p. 276

203. **B**
Phlebotomy Techniques: A Laboratory Workbook, p. 74

204. **C**
Phlebotomy Techniques: A Laboratory Workbook, p. 76

205. **B**
Phlebotomy Techniques: A Laboratory Workbook, p. 76

206. **B**
Phlebotomy Techniques: A Laboratory Workbook, p. 76

207. **A**
Phlebotomy Techniques: A Laboratory Workbook, p. 76

208. **A**
Phlebotomy Techniques: A Laboratory Workbook, p. 76

209. **A**
Phlebotomy Techniques: A Laboratory Workbook, p. 77

210. **C**
Phlebotomy Essentials, p. 379

211. **B**
Phlebotomy Essentials, p. 381

212. **C**
Phlebotomy Techniques: A Laboratory Workbook, p. 265

213. **C**
Phlebotomy Techniques: A Laboratory Workbook, p. 264; *Phlebotomy Essentials,* p. 375

214. **C**
Phlebotomy Essentials, p. 375

215. **C**
Phlebotomy Techniques: A Laboratory Workbook, p. xxi

216. **A**
Phlebotomy Essentials, p. 374

217. **A**
Phlebotomy Essentials, p. 153

218. **B**
Phlebotomy Essentials, p. 154

219. **C**
Phlebotomy Techniques: A Laboratory Workbook, p. 81

220. **C**
Phlebotomy Techniques: A Laboratory Workbook, p. 43

221. **B**
Phlebotomy Techniques: A Laboratory Workbook, pp. 86–87

222. **C**
Phlebotomy Techniques: A Laboratory Workbook, p. 87

223. **B**
Phlebotomy Techniques: A Laboratory Workbook, p. 87

224. **C**
Phlebotomy Techniques: A Laboratory Workbook, p. 87; *Phlebotomy Essentials,* p. 162

225. **D**
Phlebotomy Techniques: A Laboratory Workbook, p. 87

226. **C**
Phlebotomy Essentials, pp. 214–215

227. **C**
Phlebotomy Techniques: A Laboratory Workbook, p. 87

228. **A**
Phlebotomy Techniques: A Laboratory Workbook, p. 87

229. **C**
Phlebotomy Essentials, p. 181

230. **C**
Phlebotomy Essentials, p. 181

231. **A**
Phlebotomy Techniques: A Laboratory Workbook, p. xxi

232. **C**
Phlebotomy Essentials, p. 181

233. **A**
Phlebotomy Essentials, p. 181

234. **A**
Phlebotomy Essentials, p. 181

235. **C**
Phlebotomy Essentials, p. 181

236. **D**
Phlebotomy Essentials, p. 181

237. **B**
Phlebotomy Essentials, p. 181

238. **C**
Phlebotomy Essentials, p. 180

239. **B**
Phlebotomy Essentials, p. 181

240. **A**
Phlebotomy Essentials, p. 180

241. **B**
Phlebotomy Essentials, p. 181

242. **C**
Phlebotomy Techniques: A Laboratory Workbook, p. 88

243. **D**
Phlebotomy Techniques: A Laboratory Workbook, pp. 147–148

244. **C**
Phlebotomy Techniques: A Laboratory Workbook, p. 89

245. **C**
Phlebotomy Techniques: A Laboratory Workbook, p. 89

246. **C**
Phlebotomy Techniques: A Laboratory Workbook, pp. 144–145

247. **D**
Phlebotomy Techniques: A Laboratory Workbook, pp. 144–145

248. **D**
Phlebotomy Techniques: A Laboratory Workbook, pp. 144–145

249. **A**
Phlebotomy Techniques: A Laboratory Workbook, pp. 144–145

250. **B**
Phlebotomy Techniques: A Laboratory Workbook, pp. 144–145

251. **C**
Phlebotomy Techniques: A Laboratory Workbook, p. 144

252. **A**
Phlebotomy Techniques: A Laboratory Workbook, p. 144

253. **A**
Procedures for the Collection of Diagnostic Blood Specimens by Venipuncture, Section 6.13.3.2

254. **D**
Phlebotomy Techniques: A Laboratory Workbook, p. xxi

255. **C**
Phlebotomy Techniques: A Laboratory Workbook, p. xxi

256. **A**
Phlebotomy Techniques: A Laboratory Workbook, p. xxi

257. **C**
Phlebotomy Techniques: A Laboratory Workbook, p. 265

258. **C**
Phlebotomy Essentials, p. 381

259. **C**
Phlebotomy Essentials, p. 187

260. **A**
Phlebotomy Essentials, p. 187

261. **C**
Phlebotomy Essentials, p. 188

262. **D**
Phlebotomy Essentials, p. 188

263. **B**
Phlebotomy Essentials, p. 189

264. **B**
Phlebotomy Essentials, p. 189

265. **D**
Phlebotomy Essentials, p. 189

266. **B**
Phlebotomy Techniques: A Laboratory Workbook, p. 149

267. **B**
Phlebotomy Techniques: A Laboratory Workbook, p. 149

268. **B**
Phlebotomy Techniques: A Laboratory Workbook, p. 149

269. **B**
Phlebotomy Techniques: A Laboratory Workbook, p. 149

270. **B**
Phlebotomy Techniques: A Laboratory Workbook, p. 149

271. **B**
Phlebotomy Techniques: A Laboratory Workbook, p. 149

272. **C**
Phlebotomy Techniques: A Laboratory Workbook, p. 220

273. **D**
Phlebotomy Essentials, p. 294

274. **D**
Phlebotomy Essentials, p. 303

275. **D**
Phlebotomy Techniques: A Laboratory Workbook, p. 223

276. **A**
Phlebotomy Techniques: A Laboratory Workbook, p. 221

277. **D**
Phlebotomy Techniques: A Laboratory Workbook, p. 221

278. **B**
Phlebotomy Essentials, p. 296

279. **A**
Phlebotomy Essentials, p. 295

280. **A**
Phlebotomy Techniques: A Laboratory Workbook, p. 223

281. **C**
Phlebotomy Essentials, p. 294

282. **A**
Phlebotomy Essentials, p. 295

283. **B**
Phlebotomy Essentials, p. 296

284. **A**
Phlebotomy Essentials, p. 295

285. **B**
Phlebotomy Essentials, p. 296

286. **D**
Phlebotomy Techniques: A Laboratory Workbook, p. 223

287. **D**
Phlebotomy Techniques: A Laboratory Workbook, p. 223

288. **A**
Phlebotomy Techniques: A Laboratory Workbook, p. 223

289. **B**
Phlebotomy Essentials, p. 299

290. **B**
Phlebotomy Techniques: A Laboratory Workbook, p. 219

291. **A**
Phlebotomy Techniques: A Laboratory Workbook, p. 221

292. **D**
Phlebotomy Techniques: A Laboratory Workbook, pp. 141 and 219

293. **C**
Phlebotomy Techniques: A Laboratory Workbook, p. 219

294. **B**
Phlebotomy Techniques: A Laboratory Workbook, p. 220

295. **C**
Phlebotomy Techniques: A Laboratory Workbook, p. 220

296. **C**
Phlebotomy Techniques: A Laboratory Workbook, p. 221

297. **A**
Phlebotomy Techniques: A Laboratory Workbook, p. 224

298. **C**
Phlebotomy Techniques: A Laboratory Workbook, p. 225

299. **B**
Phlebotomy Techniques: A Laboratory Workbook, p. 221

300. **B**
Phlebotomy Techniques: A Laboratory Workbook, p. 221

301. **A**
Phlebotomy Techniques: A Laboratory Workbook, p. 222

302. **A**
Phlebotomy Techniques: A Laboratory Workbook, p. 222

303. **B**
Phlebotomy Techniques: A Laboratory Workbook, p. 222

304. **C**
Phlebotomy Handbook, Fourth Ed., p. 269

305. **C**
Phlebotomy Essentials, p. 260

306. **A**
Phlebotomy Techniques: A Laboratory Workbook, p. 265

307. **B**
Phlebotomy Techniques: A Laboratory Workbook, p. 262

308. **C**
Phlebotomy Techniques: A Laboratory Workbook, p. 163

309. **B**
Phlebotomy Techniques: A Laboratory Workbook, p. 162

310. **D**
Phlebotomy Techniques: A Laboratory Workbook, p. 162

311. **D**
Phlebotomy Techniques: A Laboratory Workbook, p. 192

312. **A**
Phlebotomy Essentials, p. 260

313. **B**
Phlebotomy Techniques: A Laboratory Workbook, p. 194

314. **C**
Phlebotomy Techniques: A Laboratory Workbook, p. 180

315. **C**
Phlebotomy Techniques: A Laboratory Workbook, p. 180

316. **B**
Phlebotomy Techniques: A Laboratory Workbook, p. 162

317. **A**
Phlebotomy Techniques: A Laboratory Workbook, p. 163

318. **B**
Phlebotomy Techniques: A Laboratory Workbook, p. 162

319. **A**
Phlebotomy Techniques: A Laboratory Workbook, p. 163

320. **D**
Phlebotomy Techniques: A Laboratory Workbook, p. 159

321. **D**
Phlebotomy Essentials, p. 165

322. **D**
Phlebotomy Techniques: A Laboratory Workbook, p. 192

323. **A**
Phlebotomy Handbook, Fourth Ed., p. 271

324. **C**
Phlebotomy Techniques: A Laboratory Workbook, p. 203

325. **B**
Phlebotomy Techniques: A Laboratory Workbook, p. 203

326. **D**
Phlebotomy Techniques: A Laboratory Workbook, p. 203

327. **B**
Phlebotomy Essentials, p. 169

328. **A**
Phlebotomy Techniques: A Laboratory Workbook, p. 211

329. **A**
Phlebotomy Techniques: A Laboratory Workbook, p. 210

330. **C**
Phlebotomy Techniques: A Laboratory Workbook, p. 46

331. **B**
Phlebotomy Techniques: A Laboratory Workbook, p. 46

332. **D**
Phlebotomy Essentials, p. 242

333. **B**
Procedures for the Collection of Diagnostic Blood Specimens by Skin Puncture, Third Ed., p. 9

334. **B**
Procedures for the Collection of Diagnostic Blood Specimens by Skin Puncture, Third Ed., p. 9

335. **C**
Phlebotomy Essentials, p. 188

336. **A**
Phlebotomy Essentials, p. 188

337. **C**
Phlebotomy Techniques: A Laboratory Workbook, p. 36

338. **A**
Phlebotomy Essentials, p. 181

339. **A**
Phlebotomy Essentials, p. 303

340. **A**
Phlebotomy Essentials, p. 303

341. **C**
Phlebotomy Essentials, p. 304

342. **A**
Phlebotomy Essentials, p. 304

343. **C**
Phlebotomy Techniques: A Laboratory Workbook, p. 220

344. **B**
Phlebotomy Techniques: A Laboratory Workbook, p. 145

345. **A**
Phlebotomy Techniques: A Laboratory Workbook, p. 144

346. **D**
Phlebotomy Techniques: A Laboratory Workbook, p. 144

347. **B**
Phlebotomy Techniques: A Laboratory Workbook, p. 136

348. **D**
Phlebotomy Techniques: A Laboratory Workbook, p. 35

349. **B**
Phlebotomy Techniques: A Laboratory Workbook, p. 35

350. **C**
Phlebotomy Techniques: A Laboratory Workbook, pp. 268–274

351. **A**
Phlebotomy Techniques: A Laboratory Workbook, p. 276

352. **B**
Phlebotomy Techniques: A Laboratory Workbook, p. 276

353. **D**
Phlebotomy Handbook, Fourth Ed., p. 23

354. **D**
Phlebotomy Techniques: A Laboratory Workbook, p. 35

355. **D**
Phlebotomy Handbook, Fourth Ed., p. 24

356. **A**
Phlebotomy Techniques: A Laboratory Workbook, p. 35

357. **A**
Phlebotomy Essentials, p. 175

358. **B**
Phlebotomy Essentials, p. 176

359. **D**
Phlebotomy Essentials, p. 381

360. **A**
Phlebotomy Essentials, p. 189

361. **D**
Phlebotomy Essentials, p. 377

362. **B**
Phlebotomy Handbook, Fourth Ed., p. 281

363. **A**
Phlebotomy Handbook, Fourth Ed., p. 270

364. **D**
Phlebotomy Techniques: A Laboratory Workbook, pp. 185–187

365. **C**
Phlebotomy Techniques: A Laboratory Workbook, p. 161

366. **D**
Phlebotomy Techniques: A Laboratory Workbook, p. 161

367. **A**
Phlebotomy Techniques: A Laboratory Workbook, p. 192

368. **D**
Phlebotomy Techniques: A Laboratory Workbook, p. 192

369. **B**
Monograph, *Blood Collection: Special Procedures* (Videotape), p. 17

370. **B**
Phlebotomy Techniques: A Laboratory Workbook, p. 193

371. **C**
Phlebotomy Techniques: A Laboratory Workbook, p. 193

372. **C**
Phlebotomy Techniques: A Laboratory Workbook, p. 194

373. **C**
Phlebotomy Techniques: A Laboratory Workbook, p. 194

374. **A**
Phlebotomy Techniques: A Laboratory Workbook, p. 194

375. **C**
Phlebotomy Handbook, Fourth Ed., p. 427

376. **A**
Phlebotomy Handbook, Fourth Ed., p. 428

377. **B**
Phlebotomy Techniques: A Laboratory Workbook, p. 193

378. **C**
Phlebotomy Techniques: A Laboratory Workbook, p. 193

379. **A**
Phlebotomy Techniques: A Laboratory Workbook, p. 193

380. **B**
Phlebotomy Techniques: A Laboratory Workbook, p. 193

381. **B**
Collection and Handling of Laboratory Specimens: A Practical Guide, p. 163

382. **C**
Collection and Handling of Laboratory Specimens: A Practical Guide, p. 166

383. **C**
Monograph, *Blood Collection: Special Procedures* (Videotape), p. 13

384. **B**
Monograph, *Blood Collection: Special Procedures* (Videotape), p. 13

385. **A**
Monograph, *Blood Collection: Special Procedures* (Videotape), p. 14

386. **B**
Monograph, *Blood Collection: Special Procedures* (Videotape), p. 14

387. **D**
Monograph, *Blood Collection: Special Procedures* (Videotape), p. 14

388. **A**
Monograph, *Blood Collection: Special Procedures* (Videotape), p. 14

389. **A**
Phlebotomy Handbook, Fourth Ed., p. 500

390. **D**
Phlebotomy Handbook, Fourth Ed., p. 501

391. **D**

392. **D**

393. **C**

394. **C**
Phlebotomy Handbook, Fourth Ed., p. 323

395. **D**
Phlebotomy Handbook, Fourth Ed., p. 325

396. **A**
Phlebotomy Handbook, Fourth Ed., p. 327

397. **C**
Phlebotomy Handbook, Fourth Ed., p. 325

398. **C**
Phlebotomy Handbook, Fourth Ed., p. 325

399. **B**
Phlebotomy Handbook, Fourth Ed., p. 331

400. **D**
Phlebotomy Essentials, p. 303

401. **A**
Phlebotomy Essentials, p. 304

402. **D**
Phlebotomy Essentials, p. 382

403. **A**
Phlebotomy Handbook, Fourth Ed., pp. 189–190

404. **D**
Phlebotomy Techniques: A Laboratory Workbook, p. 269

405. **D**
Phlebotomy Techniques: A Laboratory Workbook, p. 271

406. **D**
Phlebotomy Techniques: A Laboratory Workbook, p. 273

407. **B**
Phlebotomy Handbook, Fourth Ed., p. 22

408. **B**
Phlebotomy Essentials, p. 25

409. **C**
Phlebotomy Handbook, Fourth Ed., p. 26

410. **B**
Phlebotomy Essentials, p. 40

411. **D**
Phlebotomy Essentials, p. 34

412. **D**
Phlebotomy Essentials, p. 34

413. **B**
Phlebotomy Essentials, p. 41

414. **D**
Phlebotomy Essentials, p. 40

415. **C**
Phlebotomy Handbook, Fourth Ed., p. 333

416. **A**
Phlebotomy Handbook, Fourth Ed., p. 333

417. **B**
Phlebotomy Handbook, Fourth Ed., p. 333

418. **A**
Phlebotomy Handbook, Fourth Ed., p. 285

419. **A**
Phlebotomy Essentials, Color Plate 2

420. **D**
Phlebotomy Techniques: A Laboratory Workbook, p. 35

421. **D**
Phlebotomy Techniques: A Laboratory Workbook, p. 270

422. **B**
Phlebotomy Handbook, Fourth Ed., p. 283

423. **D**
Phlebotomy Handbook, Fourth Ed., p. 427

424. **C**
Phlebotomy Handbook, Fourth Ed., p. 427

425. **A**
Phlebotomy Workbook for the Multi-skilled Healthcare Professional, p. 363

426. **D**
Phlebotomy Workbook for the Multi-skilled Healthcare Professional, p. 363

427. **B**
Phlebotomy Workbook for the Multi-skilled Healthcare Professional, p. 363

428. **D**
Phlebotomy Workbook for the Multi-skilled Healthcare Professional, p. 363

429. **A**
Phlebotomy Workbook for the Multi-skilled Healthcare Professional, p. 362

430. **A**
Phlebotomy Workbook for the Multi-skilled Healthcare Professional, p. 364

431. **C**
Phlebotomy Workbook for the Multi-skilled Healthcare Professional, p. 364

432. **A**
Blood Collection on Filter Paper for Neonatal Screening Programs, p. 1

433. **B**
Blood Collection on Filter Paper for Neonatal Screening Programs, p. 4

434. **C**
Blood Collection on Filter Paper for Neonatal Screening Programs, p. 4

435. **D**
Blood Collection on Filter Paper for Neonatal Screening Programs, p. 4

436. **A**
Blood Collection on Filter Paper for Neonatal Screening Programs, p. 4

437. **C**
Blood Collection on Filter Paper for Neonatal Screening Programs, p. 7

438. **B**
Phlebotomy Techniques: A Laboratory Workbook, p. 172

439. **B**
Phlebotomy Workbook for the Multi-skilled Healthcare Professional, p. 333

440. **C**
Phlebotomy Workbook for the Multi-skilled Healthcare Professional, p. 342

441. **D**
Phlebotomy Workbook for the Multi-skilled Healthcare Professional, p. 342

442. **D**
Phlebotomy Workbook for the Multi-skilled Healthcare Professional, p. 342

443. **C**
Phlebotomy Workbook for the Multi-skilled Healthcare Professional, p. 343

444. **C**
Phlebotomy Essentials, Color Plate 2

445. **A**
Phlebotomy Essentials, Color Plate 2

446. **D**
Phlebotomy Techniques: A Laboratory Workbook, p. 196

447. **B**
Phlebotomy Techniques: A Laboratory Workbook, p. 194

448. **D**
Phlebotomy Techniques: A Laboratory Workbook, p. 83

449. **C**
Phlebotomy Techniques: A Laboratory Workbook, p. 35

450. **B**
Phlebotomy Techniques: A Laboratory Workbook, p. 35

451. **D**
Phlebotomy Essentials, pp. 131 and 379

452. **D**
Phlebotomy Essentials, p. 146

453. **A**
Phlebotomy Essentials, p. 140

454. **B**
Phlebotomy Essentials, p. 140

455. **C**
Phlebotomy Essentials, p. 140

456. **D**
Phlebotomy Essentials, p. 140

457. **D**
Phlebotomy Essentials, p. 141

458. **C**
Phlebotomy Handbook, Fourth Ed., p. 385

459. **D**
Phlebotomy Handbook, Fourth Ed., p. 385

460. **B**
Phlebotomy Handbook, Fourth Ed., p. 385

461. **D**
Phlebotomy Essentials, p. 139

462. **D**
Phlebotomy Essentials, p. 141

463. **B**
Phlebotomy Essentials, p. 143

464. **B**
Monograph, *Laboratory Safety and Infection Control* (Videotape), p. 8

465. **B**
Monograph, *Laboratory Safety and Infection Control* (Videotape), p. 22

466. **C**
Phlebotomy Handbook, Fourth Ed., p. 388

467. **B**
Phlebotomy Essentials, p. 131

468. **D**
Phlebotomy Handbook, Fourth Ed., p. 483

469. **B**
Phlebotomy Essentials, p. 27

470. **D**
Phlebotomy Handbook, Fourth Ed., p. 11

471. **A**
Phlebotomy Handbook, Fourth Ed., p. 11

472. **A**
Phlebotomy Handbook, Fourth Ed., p. 11

473. **D**
Phlebotomy Handbook, Fourth Ed., p. 11

474. **B**
Phlebotomy Handbook, Fourth Ed., p. 12

475. **D**
Phlebotomy Handbook, Fourth Ed., p. 12

476. **D**
Phlebotomy Handbook, Fourth Ed., p. 12

477. **A**
Phlebotomy Handbook, Fourth Ed., p. 12

478. **A**
Phlebotomy Handbook, Fourth Ed., p. 12

479. **B**
Phlebotomy Handbook, Fourth Ed., p. 13

480. **A**
Phlebotomy Handbook, Fourth Ed., p. 14

481. **B**
Phlebotomy Handbook, Fourth Ed., p. 15

482. **A**
Phlebotomy Essentials, p. 41

483. **D**
Phlebotomy Essentials, p. 42

484. **C**
Phlebotomy Essentials, p. 42

485. **B**
Phlebotomy Essentials, p. 42

486. **D**
Phlebotomy Essentials, p. 42

487. **A**
Phlebotomy Essentials, p. 41

488. **A**
Phlebotomy Handbook, Fourth Ed., pp. 18 and 19

489. **B**
Phlebotomy Techniques: A Laboratory Workbook, p. 148

490. **A**
Phlebotomy Essentials, p. 114

491. **A**
Phlebotomy Essentials, p. 378

492. **A**
Phlebotomy Handbook, Fourth Ed., p. 345

493. **A**
Phlebotomy Essentials, p. 115

494. **A**
Phlebotomy Essentials, p. 114

495. **A**
Phlebotomy Essentials, pp. 115–116

496. **D**
Phlebotomy Essentials, p. 116

497. **C**
Phlebotomy Handbook, Fourth Ed., p. 349

498. **D**
Phlebotomy Handbook, Fourth Ed., p. 350

499. **B**
Phlebotomy Handbook, Fourth Ed., p. 351

500. **C**
Phlebotomy Handbook, Fourth Ed., p. 349

501. **A**
Phlebotomy Handbook, Fourth Ed., p. 350

502. **D**
Phlebotomy Handbook, Fourth Ed., p. 351

503. **B**
Phlebotomy Essentials, p. 125

504. **B**
Phlebotomy Essentials, p. 125

505. **B**
Phlebotomy Essentials, pp. 118 and 126

506. **A**
Phlebotomy Essentials, p. 125

507. **D**
Phlebotomy Essentials, p. 379

508. **B**
Phlebotomy Essentials, pp. 121 and 131

509. **C**
Phlebotomy Essentials, p. 138

510. **A**
Phlebotomy Handbook, Fourth Ed. p. 359

511. **A**
Phlebotomy Handbook, Fourth Ed., p. 360

512. **D**
Phlebotomy Essentials, p. 118

513. **A**
Phlebotomy Essentials, p. 116

514. **B**
Phlebotomy Essentials, p. 116

515. **C**
Phlebotomy Essentials, p. 116

516. **D**
Phlebotomy Essentials, p. 117

517. **C**
Phlebotomy Essentials, p. 117

518. **B**
Phlebotomy Essentials, p. 124

519. **A**
Phlebotomy Essentials, p. 125

520. **B**
Phlebotomy Essentials, p. 125

521. **D**
Phlebotomy Essentials, p. 126

522. **B**
Phlebotomy Essentials, p. 126

523. **D**
Phlebotomy Essentials, p. 126

524. **A**
Phlebotomy Essentials, p. 126

525. **D**
Procedures in Phlebotomy, p. 54

526. **A**
Procedures in Phlebotomy, p. 54

527. **C**
Phlebotomy Essentials, p. 126

528. **D**
Phlebotomy Essentials, p. 126

529. **B**
Procedures in Phlebotomy, p. 54

530. **C**
Phlebotomy Essentials, p. 124

531. **B**
Phlebotomy Essentials, p. 126

532. **B**
Phlebotomy Essentials, p. 126

533. **B**

534. **D**
Phlebotomy Essentials, p. 122

535. **D**
Phlebotomy Essentials, p. 126

536. **A**
Phlebotomy Essentials, p. 126

537. **C**
Procedures in Phlebotomy, p. 54

538. **B**
Phlebotomy Essentials, p. 126

539. **B**
Phlebotomy Essentials, p. 126

540. **C**
Phlebotomy Essentials, p. 125

541. **B**
Phlebotomy Handbook, Fourth Ed., p. 370

542. **C**
Phlebotomy Handbook, Fourth Ed., p. 373

543. **B**
Phlebotomy Handbook, Fourth Ed., p. 373

544. **D**
Phlebotomy Handbook, Fourth Ed., p. 372

545. **B**
Phlebotomy Handbook, Fourth Ed., p. 373

546. **B**
Phlebotomy Handbook, Fourth Ed., p. 371

547. **A**
Phlebotomy Handbook, Fourth Ed., p. 371

548. **B**
Phlebotomy Essentials, p. 199

549. **C**
Phlebotomy Essentials, p. 203

550. **A**
Phlebotomy Essentials, p. 203

551. **B**
Phlebotomy Essentials, Appendix C, p. A-7

552. **A**
Phlebotomy Essentials, p. 10

553. **D**
Phlebotomy Techniques: A Laboratory Workbook, p. xvii

554. **A**
Phlebotomy Essentials, p. 119

555. **D**
Phlebotomy Techniques: A Laboratory Workbook, p. xvii

556. **A**
Phlebotomy Essentials, p. 342

557. **C**
Phlebotomy Essentials, p. 343

558. **C**
Phlebotomy Handbook, Fourth Ed., p. 405

559. **D**
Phlebotomy Handbook, Fourth Ed., p. 413

560. **A**
Phlebotomy Handbook, Fourth Ed., p. 421

561. **B**
Phlebotomy Handbook, Fourth Ed., p. 469

562. **C**
Phlebotomy Essentials, p. 342

563. **B**
Phlebotomy Handbook, Fourth Ed., p. 472

564. **A**
Phlebotomy Handbook, Fourth Ed., p. 472

565. **A**
Quality Assurance and Quality Control Procedures for Phlebotomy Techniques, *ASCP Spring Teleconference Series,* 9/14/93

566. **B**
Quality Assurance and Quality Control Procedures for Phlebotomy Techniques, *ASCP Spring Teleconference Series,* 9/14/93

567. **D**
Phlebotomy Handbook, Fourth Ed., p. 452

568. **D**
Phlebotomy Techniques: A Laboratory Workbook, p. 37

569. **D**
Phlebotomy Techniques: A Laboratory Workbook, p. 37

570. **A**
Phlebotomy Techniques: A Laboratory Workbook, p. 27

571. **D**
Phlebotomy Techniques: A Laboratory Workbook, p. 28

572. **C**
Phlebotomy Techniques: A Laboratory Workbook, p. 29

573. **D**
Phlebotomy Techniques: A Laboratory Workbook, p. 75

574. **D**
Phlebotomy Essentials, p. 9

575. **A**
Phlebotomy Essentials, p. 9

576. **A**
Phlebotomy Essentials, p. 10

577. **B**
Phlebotomy Essentials, p. 12

578. **C**
Phlebotomy Essentials, p. 378

579. **D**
Phlebotomy Handbook, Fourth Ed., p. 495

580. **B**
Phlebotomy Handbook, Fourth Ed., p. 495

581. **D**
Phlebotomy Handbook, Fourth Ed., p. 495

582. **B**
Phlebotomy Handbook, Fourth Ed., p. 505

583. **B**
Phlebotomy Essentials, pp. 376–377

584. **D**
Phlebotomy Essentials, p. 138

585. **B**
Phlebotomy Essentials, p. 335

586. **D**
Phlebotomy Techniques: A Laboratory Workbook, p. 192

587. **A**
Phlebotomy Essentials, p. 201

588. **C**
Phlebotomy Essentials, Appendix C, p. A-7

589. **B**
Phlebotomy Techniques: A Laboratory Workbook, p. 143

590. **C**
Monograph, *Laboratory Safety and Infection Control* (Videotape), p. 3

591. **A**
Monograph, *Laboratory Safety and Infection Control* (Videotape), p. 3

592. **B**
Monograph, *Laboratory Safety and Infection Control* (Videotape), p. 3

593. **D**
Monograph, *Laboratory Safety and Infection Control* (Videotape), p. 3

594. **B**
Monograph, *Laboratory Safety and Infection Control* (Videotape), p. 4

595. **B**
Monograph, *Laboratory Safety and Infection Control* (Videotape), p. 4

596. **C**
Monograph, *Laboratory Safety and Infection Control* (Videotape), p. 5

597. **B**
Monograph, *Laboratory Safety and Infection Control* (Videotape), p. 5

598. **C**
Monograph, *Laboratory Safety and Infection Control* (Videotape), p. 5

599. **C**
Phlebotomy Techniques: A Laboratory Workbook, p. 56

600. **D**
Phlebotomy Techniques: A Laboratory Workbook, p. 56

601. **B**
Phlebotomy Techniques: A Laboratory Workbook, p. 56

602. **C**
Phlebotomy Techniques: A Laboratory Workbook, p. 56

603. **A**
Phlebotomy Techniques: A Laboratory Workbook, p. 56

604. **D**
Phlebotomy Techniques: A Laboratory Workbook, p. 56

605. **B**
Phlebotomy Techniques: A Laboratory Workbook, p. 56

606. **A**
Phlebotomy Techniques: A Laboratory Workbook, p. 56

607. **A**
Phlebotomy Essentials, p. 98

608. **C**
Phlebotomy Essentials, p. 98

609. **B**
Phlebotomy Essentials, p. 98

610. **C**
Phlebotomy Essentials, p. 99

611. **B**
Phlebotomy Essentials, p. 99

612. **C**
Handbook of Phlebotomy, Third Ed., p. 58

613. **D**
Handbook of Phlebotomy, Third Ed., p. 58

614. **B**
Handbook of Phlebotomy, Third Ed., p. 59

615. **A**
Handbook of Phlebotomy, Third Ed., p. 59

616. **C**
Handbook of Phlebotomy, Third Ed., p. 60

617. **D**
Handbook of Phlebotomy, Third Ed., p. 61

618. **C**
Handbook of Phlebotomy, Third Ed., p. 54

619. **A**
Handbook of Phlebotomy, Third Ed., p. 55

620. **C**
Handbook of Phlebotomy, Third Ed., p. 55

621. **C**
Handbook of Phlebotomy, Third Ed., p. 55

622. **D**
Handbook of Phlebotomy, Third Ed., p. 55

623. **C**
Handbook of Phlebotomy, Third Ed., p. 43

624. **A**
Handbook of Phlebotomy, Third Ed., p. 43

625. **D**
Handbook of Phlebotomy, Third Ed., p. 43

626. **A**
Handbook of Phlebotomy, Third Ed., p. 43

627. **B**
Handbook of Phlebotomy, Third Ed., p. 43

628. **C**
Handbook of Phlebotomy, Third Ed., p. 43

References

Davis B. *Phlebotomy: A Client-Based Approach.* Albany, NY: Delmar Publishers; 1997.

Flynn J. *Procedures in Phlebotomy.* Philadelphia, Pa: W.B. Saunders Co; 1994.

Garza D, Becan-McBride K. *Phlebotomy Examination Review.* 2nd ed. East Norwalk, Conn: Appleton and Lange; 1993.

Garza D, Becan-McBride K. *Phlebotomy Handbook.* 4th ed. East Norwalk, Conn: Appleton and Lange; 1996.

Hoeltke L. *The Complete Textbook of Phlebotomy.* Albany, NY: Delmar Publishers; 1994.

Luebbert PP. *Laboratory Safety and Infection Control* [videotape and monograph]. Chicago, Ill: ASCP Press; 1990.

Luebbert PP. *OSHA's Bloodborne Pathogen Standard: Compliance in the Clinical Laboratory* [videotape and monograph]. Chicago, Ill: ASCP Press; 1992.

McCall R, Tankersley C. *Phlebotomy Essentials.* Philadelphia, Pa: J.B. Lippincott Company; 1993.

National Accrediting Agency for Clinical Laboratory Sciences (NAACLS). *Programs Approval Guide.* Chicago, Ill: NAACLS; 1994.

National Committee for Clinical Laboratory Standards. *Blood Collection on Filter Paper for Neonatal Screening Programs.* 2nd ed. Villanova, Pa: NCCLS; 1992.

National Committee for Clinical Laboratory Standards. *NCCLS Specimen Collection.* Villanova, Pa: NCCLS; 1992.

National Committee for Clinical Laboratory Standards. *Procedures for the Collection of Diagnostic Blood Specimens by Skin Puncture—Third Edition;* Approved Standard. NCCLS document H4-A3. (ISBN 1-56238-111-3). Villanova, Pennsylvania: NCCLS,1991.

National Committee for Clinical Laboratory Standards. *Procedures for the Collection of Diagnostic Blood Specimens by Venipuncture—Third Edition;* Approved Standard. Villanova, Pennsylvania: NCCLS, 1991.

Pendergraph G. *Handbook of Phlebotomy.* 3rd ed. Philadelphia, Pa: Lea and Febiger; 1992.

Phelan S. *Blood Collection: Special Procedures* [videotape and monograph]. Chicago, Ill: ASCP Press; 1991.

Phelan S. *Blood Collection: The Pediatric Patient* [videotape and monograph]. Chicago, Ill: ASCP Press; 1990.

Phelan S. *Phlebotomy Techniques: A Laboratory Workbook.* Chicago, Ill: ASCP Press; 1993.

Slockbower JM, Blumenfeld TA. *Collection and Handling of Laboratory Specimens: A Practical Guide*. Philadelphia Pa: J.B. Lippincott Co; 1983.

Strasinger S, Di Lorenzo M. *Phlebotomy Workbook for the Multiskilled Healthcare Professional*. Philadelphia, Pa: F.A. Davis Co; 1996.